THE

Red

JOURNAL

Track your period,
sync with your cycle,
and unlock your
monthly
superpowers

LISA LISTER

HAY HOUSE

Carlsbad, California • New York City
London • Sydney • New Delhi

This Journal Belongs to

Published in the United Kingdom by:
Hay House UK Ltd, The Sixth Floor, Watson House,
54 Baker Street, London W1U 7BU
Tel: +44 (0)20 3927 7290; Fax: +44 (0)20 3927 7291; www.hayhouse.co.uk

Published in the United States of America by:
Hay House Inc., PO Box 5100, Carlsbad, CA 92018-5100
Tel: (1) 760 431 7695 or (800) 654 5126
Fax: (1) 760 431 6948 or (800) 650 5115; www.hayhouse.com

Published in Australia by:
Hay House Australia Ltd, 18/36 Ralph St, Alexandria NSW 2015
Tel: (61) 2 9669 4299; Fax: (61) 2 9669 4144; www.hayhouse.com.au

Published in India by:
Hay House Publishers India, Muskaan Complex, Plot No.3, B-2,
Vasant Kunj, New Delhi 110 070
Tel: (91) 11 4176 1620; Fax: (91) 11 4176 1630; www.hayhouse.co.in

A catalogue record for this book is available from the British Library.

ISBN: 978-1-78817-552-4

Interior images: diagrams on pages 7, 26, and 'Your Cycle Wheel' on page 47 and repeated throughout, all by Jade Ho Design.

Contents

Introduction

The *Red Journal* is your bloody brilliant way to get to know yourself better by charting your menstrual cycle.

Why would you want to do that?

Well, there's a gazillion reasons, but if you didn't know already, the act of regularly charting and tracking your menstrual cycle is a major power move in understanding why you do, think, and act the way you do, and it's the key to unlocking your own set of unique-to-you monthly superpowers.

Once your monthly superpowers are unlocked and activated, you can use them to support you, to build a relationship of trust with your body and its wisdom, and you also get to create a bloody amazing life that's in complete sync with your cycle.

It's no secret that many of us have probably, at one time or another, cursed our period, found it annoying, have been shamed for it, have been embarrassed by it and/or generally found it rather bloody inconvenient. Yet we experience roughly between 350 to 500 menstrual cycles in our lifetime and each one has the potential for us to listen to our body and get better acquainted with ourselves, so it makes total sense for us to get to know our flow.

As you move through each of the phases, you'll notice that, each month, you experience your life through the lens of the phase that you're currently in. In each phase, you feel, act and show up to life very differently. When you chart your cycle, you'll realize, really quite quickly, that your menstrual cycle is way more than just a biological process; it's a cycle of ever-changing spiritual, emotional, hormonal, creative energy that becomes a map of YOUR landscape throughout the menstrual month.

Can you see how knowing this information will help you to plan and organize your life? Charting and tracking your cycle also becomes a super-supportive self-care tool. It gives you the opportunity to recognize what you actually need and want in each phase (from the food you eat to the exercise you take, from the perfume you wear to how you like to orgasm). You'll start to recognize that, in each phase, your list of feel-good requirements are totally different.

The Red Journal is a know-yourself-better space to chart your moods, your feels, and your energy levels. You can take note of when you're most chatty and available for conversations, when you're feeling sexy (and also when you want to stab your partner in the eye because they're breathing too heavily—yes, that's a personal observation from day 25 of my own Red Journal: real talk). There's also space for you to review and reflect on each cycle.

Let what you discover be the start of an incredible relationship with yourself. One where you have self-knowing, agency, and the power to create a bloody brilliant life.

Big love,

Lisa x

Know Your Flow

Knowing your body, your tendencies, your patterns is... EVERYTHING. It's what I call cyclic intelligence and it's THE. GOOD. STUFF.

All the information you'll *ever* need to know about yourself can be witnessed as you move through your menstrual cycle.

In each phase, you have access to insight, codes, and wisdom that can be used to understand and enhance your life, and as you move from one phase to the next, your cycle offers up an amazing opportunity for you to align and live in sync with this wisdom.

Yep, our bodies are deeply tuned in to the cycles of nature, the moon, the elements, the cosmos, except we've been conditioned to ignore our cyclic nature. Instead, we multi-task, we feel like we need to do it ALL in order to be good or successful, we're told to trust external teachers and voices rather than our own body and its wisdom. In the process, we've cultivated a very linear, straight-line, goal-orientated existence. One where we've lost connection to the power that we experience when we have a deep awareness and knowing of who we are through the lens of the menstrual cycle.

`Cycle awareness = self awareness`

`Self awareness = power and agency`

Cycle awareness

Previously the exclusive terrain of those who wanted to get pregnant, cycle awareness is now a practical AND beautiful way for anyone who wants to get curious about why they do the things they do to learn what's *actually* going on in their body, and how they can work with their cyclic nature and not against it.

How it works:

- You know where you're at in your cycle at any given moment.
- You pay attention to your feels, your body sensations, and your hormonal changes.
- You respond, not react, to what you discover.
- You begin to cultivate a fierce, loving, and ever-evolving relationship with yourself.

Now, if you've ever experienced any pain, discomfort, embarrassment, blame, or shame regarding your menstrual cycle, this may feel like something that is NEVER going to happen.

I hear you, that's exactly how I felt.

After years of misdiagnosis and bleeding more days than I wasn't, after wishing daily for a different body or for someone just to remove my womb already, I was told I had endometriosis and polycystic ovary syndrome (PCOS). At the time, I was grateful for a diagnosis. FINALLY.

I was then told, moments later by a dude in a white coat, that I had zero chance of having kids so they may as well *"whip it out"* (he was referring to my womb), and I'm not going to lie, I was I tempted. Unfortunately, this doctor's response is NOT uncommon. I hear from clients weekly in response to their menstrual and sexual health that they've been told, *"There's nothing we can do, you're going to have to live with the pain, heavy bleeding, or no periods, or obviously we can take it out."* Many of my clients have been prescribed the pill as a way to "manage" their symptoms instead of working with them, the way that I do, to get to the root cause.

So why did I decide against the "whip out" solution?

I share the full story in my book *Code Red* but, ultimately, I had a deeper knowing that there had to be more to it. There had to be more choices than simply taking synthetic hormones, painkillers or having my reproductive organs "whipped out".

So I gave myself six months and I started to chart my cycle (something I thought only people who wanted to get pregnant did), and in the process, I discovered...

- my landscape
- my terrain
- my magic
- my power

When you get familiar with yourself through cycle awareness, you:

- begin to pick up on your body's cues (even the more subtle ones)
- recognize that the pain and discomfort you experience are in fact a message that something deeper is going on for you and is wanting to be addressed
- become more responsive to your physical, emotional, and spiritual needs
- find that your *Red Journal* (and all the cycle intel you gather in it) becomes your very own self-help book and life coach

- are able to trust yourself to make smarter decisions and better choices, and live your life in ways that feel creative, juicy, supportive, and nourishing.

When you know why you do the things you do and why you act a certain way at certain times of the month, you begin to breathe a little easier, you're less hard on yourself and, despite what you may have previously been told, you realize that you're not crazy. You realize that you're not consistent either, you're in fact cyclic and that? Well, that is a GOOD thing.

FYI: Being consistent is an outdated, societal construct designed to keep us "doing" and in action, but it's simply not sustainable to stay one way indefinitely. I mean, you CAN, but the chances are you'll end up exhausted, depleted and burnt out. In fact, not honoring your natural and cyclical rhythms can create subtle, yet persistent states of depression, anxiety, and exhaustion, which ultimately lead to you never actually living a full and vital life.

> When we understand, acknowledge and
> accept our cyclic nature, we understand,
> acknowledge and accept ourselves.
> Hurrah for THAT.

So, let's crack the spine on this journal (it always makes writing in a brand-new book so much easier, doesn't it?! Go on, I dare you!) and let's get to know your flow.

It will transform your relationship with your body, with work, with money, with Mumma Nature and with others.

> If you let it, knowing your flow will
> change your bloody life.

A Cyclic Health Check

Many of us have been told that our menstrual cycle is the five to seven(ish) days that we actually bleed.

NOT true.

Your time of the month?

It's ALL bloody month.

In fact, virtually every part of your body is affected during every stage of your menstrual cycle—pulse rate, blood pressure, body temperature, even how many times you need to pee and poo are affected, and you've got your hormones to thank for that.

 Estrogen

 Testosterone

 Progesterone

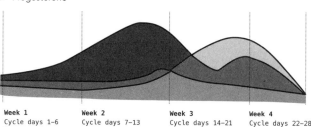

Week 1	Week 2	Week 3	Week 4
Cycle days 1–6	Cycle days 7–13	Cycle days 14–21	Cycle days 22–28
Menstruation	Pre-ovulation	Ovulation	Pre-menstruation
Winter/New Moon	Spring/Waxing Moon	Summer/Full Moon	Fall/Waning Moon

Every cycle, you go through a complex series of hormonal changes which stimulate a ton of different reactions and responses in your body. Charting these can provide you with some serious data about your health. In fact, the menstrual cycle has been called, by doctors and science people, the fifth vital sign.

Know your cycle, know your health, know yourself.

If you're experiencing an "average" cycle, you'll ovulate around 14(ish) days after the first day of your period.

HEADS UP: when I say "average", I mean what's considered "normal". The WHOLE POINT of tracking and charting your cycle is to find out what is YOUR "average" and "normal", okay? A friend of yours may love her ovulation phase, she may be super-switched on, really productive and feel sassy and sexy during that phase, while you, on the other hand, may experience the worst kind of cramps, feel completely over-exposed and like you want to hide indefinitely for your entire ovulation phase. This could be how it is for you, or the ovulation pain you experience could be a signal that something's up or it could be that you're simply feeling this way, THIS cycle, because maybe life events are a little overwhelming for you right now.

That's why tracking and charting is my favorite way to witness my OWN personal cyclic experience. When I chart, I can see where I may be experiencing challenges in my cycle, I can see (and you will too as you fill the pages of your *Red Journal* each cycle) if that's happening for me every cycle, and I can then see what, if any, changes I may need to make, help I need to seek, action I need to take in order to feel as vital, juicy, and creative as possible.

Yep, that's the point of our cycle. It's a cycle of creation.

What you decide to create, however, is totally up to you—if it's possible for you (and if you want to, of course), that creation might be an actual life, it might be extra energy, a piece of art, good health, an exciting new project, or you might want to launch a business— the deal is, when you know your cycle, when you follow its clues and cues, you become nourished and fecund, and you can create ANYTHING.

Feeling juicy?

Let's get familiar with your juices.

Yep, from around day 8-ish of your cycle, your cervical fluid is a visual way to track where you're at and your 'down-there' health. It's clever like that.

When the fluid is slippery, stretchy and egg-white-y (technical term), sound the klaxon: you're ovulating. Basically, immediately prior to and during ovulation, this is your cervix letting you know that you are a powerhouse of creative possibility.

Estrogen is at its peak, the follicle with your egg inside it is at its largest and is letting you know that you can make a baby OR facilitate the creation of... well, just about bloody anything. If you don't want to make a baby when your vag is making slippery egg-white fluid, you DEFFO need to use a barrier method, because this is the good stuff. It's the stuff of sperm-y dreams. When you're ovulating, you're magnetic, your aura stretches to 26 feet (that's an exaggeration, but y'know, it's big), you're a manifesting queen, capable of creating ANYTHING with, and from, your yoni-verse.

Aren't we bloody incredible?

Basically, ovulation is a signal point that you're at the "middle" of your cycle.

When cervical fluid becomes milkier, more sticky, and less stretchy, it's a sign that ovulating is over and you're moving into your premenstrual phase.

Period blood consistency

Now, some people get totally ick-ed out when I suggest they get familiar with the color, consistency, and texture of their actual period blood, but the appearance of your menstrual blood is a super-helpful way to check-in with your hormonal health.

You can use the color and texture of your blood as an indicator as to which hormones are in, and out, of balance for you.

MASSIVE CAVEAT: I am NOT a doctor, I'm a menstrual health practitioner and what I share here is simply a guide to support you as you make informed decisions about *your* menstrual health.

A "healthy" period

A "healthy" period will most often be a cranberry-red color and jelly-like in consistency for the majority of your bleed.

Brown and thin

If you experience a mostly brown and thin consistency on most of the days that you bleed each month, there's a chance you have low progesterone levels and what you're seeing when you bleed is old, oxidized blood that may have been stagnating for a few cycles.

Dark, thick, and clotty

If you experience a thick and clotty darker bleed, this may be a sign of too much estrogen and you may also experience a longer bleed and lots of pain and cramps too. Those who experience endometriosis and fibroids may have a flood flow similar in consistency to this.

Pink and barely there

If your bleed is barely there and is more pink than it is red for the majority of your bleed, this could mean your estrogen levels are too low. This is the kind of bleed you may experience if you're deficient in certain nutrients, or have burnout or adrenal fatigue.

None of this is bad or wrong, but tracking it, seeing if there's a difference in consistency, texture, and color each cycle, can help you to see exactly what you're experiencing and learn how you can support yourself and your hormonal health.

For example, when I've been particularly stressed and anxious during a cycle, I notice that my menstruation phase will become a lot shorter and has a tendency to become really light, but this is NOT my pattern. When the stress and anxiety lessen, my menstruation returns to five days and it became darker in color.

Getting familiar with your blood makes it easier to understand what might be going on and to seek the support you need.

A health professional who specializes in hormonal health will be able to work with you and your entire cyclic experience, and that will be much easier to do if you've been tracking your cycle and have intel to share.

Stress and mental health

Stress *will* hijack your hormones. Actual fact.

When your body is stressed, your cortisol production rises, your progesterone levels lower and it means that estrogen is going to dominate. We do NOT want that. Why?

Because you become inflamed, you sleep less, you become grumpy and potentially really bloody irritable. It also means that your actual period itself might be extra crampy and painful.

As you track, take notes of times in your cycle when you're getting stressed or when you're not sleeping. Maybe you get really stressed in week 2 of your cycle, and maybe as you track, you start to recognize that you take on too much at work and say "yes" when you actually mean "no" and so you stay up later than you'd like, or you're worrying about whether you'll get it done, so you can't sleep.

When we see the patterns reveal themselves, we can see what we need to do so that we don't become as stressed. Maybe we need to say "no" more, maybe we need to make a promise to ourselves that we work no later than 7 p.m., perhaps we need to schedule in a morning breath and movement class so that we're less likely to feel so stressed throughout the day.

Dr Jolene Brighten, author of *Beyond the Pill*, suggests considering the following factors to support hormonal health during your cycle:

Magnesium

Magnesium inhibits prostaglandins—you know, those little hormone-like substances that like to make those cramps so bad? Yeah, that's the stuff I'm talking about. If you're someone who has headaches that come along with your period, magnesium can work wonders.

Typically, I would recommend in my clinic that women begin with 150–300mg of magnesium nightly. Then increase to anywhere from 300–600mg the week before their period.

Tumeric

Turmeric is an anti-inflammatory and supports healthy liver detox. It's also fantastic for gut health, which is an essential foundational piece in creating hormonal balance. Turmeric can reduce pain-driving prostaglandins and supports healthy estrogen levels.

Blood sugar balance

If you experience irregular periods this is definitely essential for you. Make sure you're eating regular meals throughout the day. Include fat and protein with each of your meals as this will help with your insulin and blood sugar levels so that the rest of your hormones can get back into balance.

Things to look for when charting

Irregularity

I get asked about irregular periods ALL. THE. TIME.

We've been told that our period 'should' be 28 days, but what I've found, as a menstrual health practitioner, is that it really does vary from person to person and doesn't always mean that there's something wrong if yours is longer or shorter.

What matters, and this is DEFINITELY a reason to chart, is whether they're irregularly irregular. What I mean by this is, if your cycle is 23 days long for a consecutive amount of months (and you'll be able to confirm that by tracking), then that may be YOUR regular. If your cycle is 39 days long, and it's 39 days EVERY cycle, that too may be YOUR regular.

Now, if you have NO IDEA when your period is showing up and one month it's 22 days and the next 45, this unpredictability can be a sign that something is going on that needs attention.

My suggestion? Chart for at least three to six months, take notes of any patterns that you see emerging and seek support either from your doctor or a menstrual health practitioner.

Pain

Guess what? Having your period is NOT meant to be painful.

I know, right? Yes, there's definitely a chance that your uterus doubling in size may cause a few cramps or two, but it should *not* be taking you out for entire days each month and you absolutely should *not* need to take ALL the painkillers simply to get you through a day. The reasons as to *why* you're experiencing pain can be dependent on *many* things—but do know that if you are experiencing pain, please don't "put up with it". There are lots of lifestyle, nutritional, psychological, and supplement support options you can work with to help ease it.

One of my clients experienced THE worst mood swings in the week before she bled and then, when she did bleed, it was so painful she couldn't leave the house. By tracking her cycle, making a note of her productivity and work hours along with what she was eating, it was clear that she was pushing herself REALLY hard in the first half of her cycle. She was burning the candle at both ends, eating takeouts and chocolate and overworking, which led to increased estrogen and to inflammation in both her body and emotions during her premenstrual phase. The estrogen dominance was then causing cramps and heavy bleeding during menstruation.

She made some lifestyle changes, she reorganized her work schedule and we found magnesium was a fierce friend in helping her overcome the cramps and heavy bleeding.

Remember, while I may be a menstrual health practitioner, I'm not YOUR menstrual health practitioner, so make sure you're receiving the right support for *your* needs.

Missing periods

Sometimes we get so busy with living life that we don't actually notice when we miss a period. This is why tracking can really be useful, because missing periods, especially if it's for more than three months, is a "thing". It's called Amenorrhea and it could mean that you're:

- perimenopausal
- just come off of birth control
- pregnant
- experiencing high amounts of stress
- OR a variety of other possible reasons.

Premenstrual syndrome

PMS is something we're told is just simply part of having a menstrual cycle.

Wrong.

It shows up for many of us (but not exclusively) who are living a fast-paced life and have difficulty in resting. Obviously, as with everything I share here, there may be many reasons as to why we experience PMS, and because we're told that we just have to "put up with it" we probably ignore, push aside, or medicate the physical and emotional symptoms that can occur directly after ovulation and before you start to bleed. Those symptoms may include: feeling irritable and tired, craving fatty, sugary food, anxiety, lots of tears, lack of interest in anything sex related (and potentially many, many more).

Science-y people suggest that PMS happens after ovulation because when your body finds out it's not pregnant, estrogen and progesterone levels drop drastically. PMS symptoms and feelings seem to go away within a few days after a woman's period starts as hormone levels begin rising again. One of the most radical things I've experienced with my clients when they track their cycle is that they are able to find the hot spots and trigger points within their cycle that can activate their PMS. Then, over a few months of making oftentimes really quite small changes to their lifestyle, the symptoms lessen and in some cases can disappear entirely.

Premenstrual dysphoric disorder

Now, I don't often speak about this, but I'm doing it to take away any stigma or shame that I know clients have often felt when sharing their own experience of PMDD with me.

I myself was diagnosed with premenstrual dysphoric disorder a few years ago.

Yep, despite knowing EVERYTHING I know about our cyclic nature, I genuinely thought I was going mad and had to seek help. For me, PMDD presents as my wanting to physically scratch myself out of my skin (and sometimes I scratch so hard I actually bleed). My sensitivity is so heightened in my premenstrual phase that it feels like I'm wearing my nervous system on the outside and that someone is constantly rubbing sandpaper over my entire body. My thoughts can get really dark, really quickly, and I can spiral from 1 to totally-out-of-control in a heartbeat.

In *Code Red*, from a more psycho-spiritual perspective, I speak about how our premenstrual phase is where our intuition and senses are heightened, so it makes sense that we are supersensory here, but for those who experience PMDD, the intensity of feeling can feel overwhelming and *too much*.

It can cause physical symptoms like cramps, joint pain, and bloating, along with severe irritability, depression, and/or anxiety in the week or two before your period starts, with symptoms usually going away two to three days after your period starts.

NOTE: I share all of this not to put a label on my, or others', cyclic symptoms and experience. I don't subscribe to labels, medical or otherwise, but what I personally have found is that knowing there's a science-y term, along with data to support the things that would otherwise make me (and others) think we're actually mad in regards to our menstrual cycle, really bloody helps in being able to work with the symptoms and not become a victim to them.

ANOTHER NOTE: I'm sure you've noticed by now, but there is sadly *not* a one-size-fits-all diagnosis or solution for the many, many kinds of menstrual and reproductive discomfort or dis-ease that many of us experience. How we experience it, and therefore what will be necessary in order to ease it and support it, will be dependent on so many factors—our body, our nervous system, our lifestyle, our ability to rest and relax, the relationships we're in, our spiritual beliefs... the list is endless.

This is why we track our cycle (one of the many reasons, at least): because, by doing so, we collect data on ourselves. We bring awareness to the body, and we take notes. We get curious about ourselves, and when something isn't right we can take our findings to a health practitioner, and instead of handing over our power and asking to be "fixed", we can seek support and healing from a place of agency and self-knowledge.

ONE MORE NOTE: While I can support you in working with the foundations of your hormonal menstrual wellness, I predominantly support the psychological, somatic, and spiritual experience of the menstrual cycle. Women I love and trust who talk about the menstrual cycle as the fifth vital sign and who know everything there is to know about hormonal health are:

Dr Jolene Brighten—author of *Beyond the Pill*
Dr Christiane Northrup—author of *Women's Bodies, Women's Wisdom*
Alissa Vitti—author of *WomanCode*

It's a Phase

The moon and menstrual phases

Now, just like the moon, your menstrual cycle follows roughly a 29-day cycle and, in the same way that the moon waxes and wanes, so do you.

Each month, we take a trip through the light and dark part of ourselves—in many indigenous tribes, the word for "moon" and "menstruation" are interchangeable, and that's because most societies have, at one time or another, understood the link between the menstrual cycle and the moon.

The moon is the primary symbol for feminine energy and she takes about 29 days to circle the Earth, roughly the same amount of time as the "average" woman's menstrual cycle. Both have energetic phases that hold medicine and intel that can support us as we navigate our experience.

To understand our own cyclic nature, we can turn to the moon and feel the energetics of each of her phases on the collective—by that I mean, how she affects us all.

From new, the moon grows and becomes bright and full—this half of the cycle is masculine, out-there, "doing" energy.

Then, as she begins to decrease in size and move back towards the darkness, this half of the cycle is feminine, inward-facing energy.

Waxing Moon

Full Moon

Waning Moon

Dark Moon

Waxing Moon

When the Moon is "waxing," she's getting larger in the sky, moving from the New Moon toward the Full Moon. This is a time of growth, a time to start new projects, meet new people, take risks, conceptualize ideas, to play and attract new love in your life.

Full Moon

When the Moon is full, she forms a perfect silvery sphere of gorgeousness in the sky. This is a time for those ideas you conceptualized during the Waxing Moon to manifest. It's a time to be seen. You may feel extra frisky and your senses may be heightened in this phase. At the Full Moon, feelings and emotions are amplified and illuminated—*everything* is seen—so if you're an introvert or you're hyper-sensitive, this phase can often feel a little "too much". What this phase does do, however, is let everything be felt and seen—so you can use the Moon phases that follow to edit and release what's for keeps and what's no longer necessary.

Waning Moon

Once the Moon has reached its fullness, the Waning Moon decreases in size as it moves back toward the dark of the Moon. The energy of this phase is best used to edit, clear out, break bad habits or bad addictions, and end bad relationships. In this phase of the Moon, your intuition is heightened and your tolerance and patience levels may be lower than usual.

Dark Moon/New Moon

This is when the moon is directly between the Earth and the Sun and is therefore hidden. The Dark Moon occurs in the days leading up to when the moon becomes new. This can feel quite intense, and you may feel the need to reschedule dates or plans in favor of alone time, meditation, and silence. The Dark Moon can also cause your feelings to seem like they're *over-feel-y*, so you might notice that you binge on food, TV, and social media to try to numb out. When the moon turns new, however, set your intentions for the cycle ahead.

The wise women before us were in total sync with the moon; they knew that our menstrual cycle is highly affected by the moon's movement. Their blood and hormonal cycle followed the moon's ebb and flow; as the cycle waxed from New Moon to Full Moon, estrogen levels increased, leading to supercharged fertility when the moon was at her fullest, roundest, and most abundant. From Full Moon to New Moon, the waning half of the cycle, progesterone dominated and led to the release of blood at the Dark Moon.

Today, most of us are totally out of sync with the moon's cycles. We get so busy in our daily lives that for the most part we ignore the cyclic changes of Mumma Nature—the seasons, the moon, the ebb and flow of the sea—all of which are indicative as to how we could be living.

One of the questions I get asked most is *"How do I sync my cycle to the moon?"* By which the person usually means, how can I make it so that, like the wise women who went before, I ovulate with the Full Moon and bleed with the Dark Moon.

While this *is* possible, please know that it's NOT necessary.

From blue light to street lights, to the amount of contraception in our water system, it's rare that any of us actually bleed in sync with the moon anymore, so despite what you may have been told, you really don't need to sync your cycle with the moon because, guess what? It already is.

Whichever moon phase you bleed in (and you'll notice this will change depending on what's being called up and through you to respond to, and work with, during the years that you bleed) holds its own power and magic for what you need to receive right now.

If you bleed during a Waxing Moon

You're being called to use your menstruation phase to explore, get curious, and make new discoveries about yourself and the world. Read books that hold teachings you've meant to read but haven't got around to, or listen to podcasts that inspire you. This is a time to grow and play, taste different foods, take a left when you'd usually take a right. Dare to try new things and you'll care less about failing if you bleed during a Waxing Moon.

If you bleed during a Full Moon

You're being called to share your work, medicine, and experience with the collective. Bleeding at the Full Moon is a call to use the vitality and potent power of the Full Moon along with the release of menstruation to bring something into being; to create, birth, and nourish outwardly, for the world. It will be no surprise that right now, many women will be bleeding with the Full Moon because they're being called to act and create in response to political and environmental situations. Their work here is to turn rage into creative action.

If you bleed during a Waning Moon

You're being called to tend to the blooms and manifestations of the previous Full Moon. It's an invitation to use the information you've opened up to receiving during your bleedtime (I'll explain later, but you're a divination rod for Source when you bleed), to help you get geeky with the details, really stabilize and solidify already-existing conditions, and verify the knowledge that will help to develop plans and projects.

If you bleed during a Dark Moon/New Moon

You're being called inward. To nourish yourself FULLY. Your dream time will be extra potent, so be sure to make lots of notes because when you bleed during this phase of the Moon, you have one foot in this world and one foot in the great void: the cosmic womb. You have access to all that's been and all that's to come—it's pretty wild. It's a good time to be still, to be in silence, and to let your wisest self be your guide so that you can set clear intentions for the cycle ahead.

How it is for you may be different from how it is for me, and that's OK. As you chart your cycle, take a look at the phase of the Moon and then turn your attention to how you feel. The menstrual cycle and Moon connection can hold a LOT of intel and wisdom for you.

Why Track Your Cycle?

There are SO many reasons to track your cycle:

- You'll know when your period is actually coming. No more surprise I-need-to-get-to-the-loo-quick situations.

- You'll know when you're ovulating too, so if you don't want to get pregnant, you'll know when to use a barrier method. (Again no surprises—knowledge is power, right?)

- You'll see how long your cycle is, if it's regular or irregular. You'll see how long your bleed is too.

- You'll know when you might feel bloated, powerful, tired or full of energy.

- You'll know when your body is out of whack.

- You'll be able to access and increase the power and badass-ery that lies in knowing and trusting your body.

Whatever your current menstrual-cycle situation, whether you're on the pill, your cycle is irregular, you're perimenopausal, you've got PCOS, endometriosis, or fibroids (or any of the other gazillion reasons why you might find your period painful, annoying and like you'd rather do anything besides ACTUALLY PAYING ATTENTION to it), charting your cycle will help you to connect to yourself, exactly where you're at right now.

Let it be an experiment. An opportunity to gain body awareness, to be present with what's going on for YOU. When I first started sharing about menstrual-cycle awareness, I was always quite concerned that charting your cycle might be seen as yet another "protocol" or "system", another way to measure how "well" you're doing at life. Please know that it's NOT.

Charting your cycle is a way to get to know what's going on for YOU. So don't read what's shared here, or in *Code Red*, and think, "Well, my cycle's not like that, so I must be doing something wrong." You're charting and tracking and journaling to get to know yourself better through the cyclic experience.

I often hear: "Oh, I bleed with the New Moon so that means I'm in sync with the moon cycle, right?" Or, "I don't feel super-creative or chatty at ovulation: in fact, it often feels too bright and too much—does that mean I'm doing ovulation wrong?" The answer is "no" to both of them.

We chart to learn as much as we can about ourselves, NOT to find yet more ways to beat ourselves up, shame or prove ourselves. In fact, the reason why I'm so passionate about encouraging you to track is so that we can undo some of that shame-and-blame training that we've been subjected to and create a place of safety and trust in your body, because self-knowledge = power.

How and What to Chart

I've been charting my cycle for many, many years now, and each cycle I learn a little bit more about myself, and the more I learn, the more I'm able to fully own my powers, care for myself without fear or guilt, and live my life in ways that feel totally aligned and meaningful to me. Of course, you could download a period-tracking app on your phone and fill in the basic details, but the *real* magic happens when you journal.

There are cycles that map the most auspicious times for everything in life. We are fortunate enough to have an internal map—the menstrual cycle—that gives us directions for the most promising and potent times for everything we do.

Unfortunately, Western culture has deemed this inner guidance system obsolete, and has reprogrammed us to follow the timing of a modern prescribed calendar, a calendar operating seven days a week, as opposed to following the timing of our own bodies in accordance with the timing of nature.

So, let's keep it really simple. The cycles of womanhood, the seasons, the elements, the moon, and your menstrual cycle can all be mapped as follow:

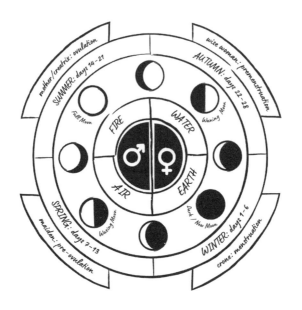

Air	Waxing moon	Pre-Ovulation	Spring	Maiden
Fire	Full Moon	Ovulation	Summer	Mumma/ Creatrix
Water	Waning Moon	Premenstruation	Autumn	Wise Woman
Earth	Dark /New Moon	Menstruation	Winter	Crone

Through **pre-ovulation/Waxing Moon/spring** and **ovulation/Full Moon/summer**, our energy is masculine. We become powered by the sun, we're outwards-focused and, like the moon as it moves from waxing to full, we are growing, we are taking in a really big breath, and expanding outwardly.

Then, when we reach **premenstrual/Waning Moon/autumn** and **menstruation/Dark Moon/winter**, we start to turn inwards, our energy is less "out there" and this is a much more feminine energy, it's that deep release we experience when we exhale.

So the inhalation is masculine, filling us up with go-for-it, take-action energy, while the exhalation is feminine and is a deep release, a time to slow down and surrender inwards—and this beautiful yin-and-yang exchange, this masculine and feminine dance, is happening in our breath, in the cycles of the moon, in the seasons, and in our menstrual cycle.

Getting to know your menstrual cycle and the cycles of Mumma Nature and the moon is a map for creating a life in sync with the feminine rhythms of nature that we're each connected to, and offers up the possibility of drawing strength and superpowers from each phase.

Pre-ovulation

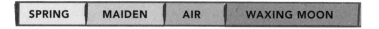

SPRING	MAIDEN	AIR	WAXING MOON

You've just bled, and now there's potential to start again. A rebirth.

We are SO lucky (I know it might not always feel like it) that each month, just like when spring arrives, we get the opportunity to start over. Pre-ovulation is the first phase of your cycle and usually begins around day 6 or 7, and carries on all the way through to day 13. (Obviously, this will vary depending on the length of your cycle and it may take a few months of charting to really start to see where each phase begins and ends for you, but that's part of your very own exploration.)

So, in the seven to ten days after your bleed, you will start to come out of your winter-like cocoon and a steady increase in estrogen will boost your brain's serotonin levels, which leads to an increase in energy and enthusiasm for… well, just about everything, and you'll feel a lot more upbeat than you did in your previous bleed days. Hurrah. You may want to spend time with friends, dance, start a new class, and learn a new skill. Words come easily and you're articulate, so if you've got a big presentation or an important call to make, definitely do it in this phase of your cycle.

With each cycle, your pre-ovulation is a brand-new page, an opportunity to write a new chapter in the ever-unfolding story of you, and like Dorothy in *The Wizard of Oz*, you get to set off on an adventure that will always lead you back home to yourself. Except, unlike Dorothy, your path isn't yellow, it's blood red. (And of course, the ruby-red shoes are optional, but come on, who wouldn't want a pair of sparkly ruby-red shoes?!)

Ovulation

SUMMER	MUMMA/CREATRIX	FIRE	FULL MOON

At ovulation, a tiny egg has been released from one of your two ovaries. This is the time you are most likely to get pregnant—you've been warned. Wink.

This is the second phase of your cycle and usually begins around day 13, continuing all the way through to day 21, during which time it may feel like you have a neon sign above your head flashing: 'I'm hot-to-trot, come and get me!' and that's because... you're ovulating.

Ovulation happens when estrogen and testosterone reach their highest peaks during your cycle. This means that the optimism, confidence, personal power and the "doing" mentality that have all been growing since day 1 of your cycle are now peaking too. Oh yes, to quote many social media memes: "You're high-vibe, baby!"

Like the Full Moon when she is ripe and has reached her full potential, during ovulation you become your most full and your most present.

It's a time when you become pregnant with life. Literally, in some cases. Even if you're not, you'll definitely be feeling much more nurturing, passionate and compassionate at this time. You may experience a strong need to reach out and to work, collaborate, make out with and to generally be with people. Even the most introverted amongst us may find it much more easier to be with, and around, people during ovulation than at any other time in our cycle.

Premenstruation

AUTUMN	WISE WOMAN	WATER	WANING MOON

This is the third phase of your cycle and if your egg wasn't fertilized during ovulation, from roughly day 23 through to your bleed, you will experience a withdrawal by all three of the following hormones—estrogen, testosterone, and progesterone.

Basically, we've been going full speed in the first half of our cycle, and it's here, in premenstruation, that we realize that we're not ACTUALLY Queen of EVERYTHING.

And that is not always a welcome discovery. Our tolerance level is much lower than it would have been in the previous part of our cycle—you've got dropping hormone levels to thank for *that*—and your energy levels begin to drop too, so you physically can't (and more importantly, shouldn't) do as much as you were doing previously. It's your body's cue to sl-o-o-o-o-w down. Until now, your attention has been outward-focused but this is the time to start bringing that attention inwards towards your own needs and requirements, letting go of what's no longer required, editing your life so that you can really receive *exactly* what you need.

You may find yourself getting more mad than usual at a partner or a child for leaving their dirty clothes on the landing.

It's a time when we can really tap into our inner wisdom, vision and intuition, *and* it's when our inner critic may show up louder than usual, so be warned.

FYI: It's also when I have the sharpest tongue and no filter, so I try, when possible, to not enter into too much social interaction at this time, as my sensitivity is heightened while my tolerance levels are super-low in the premenstrual phase.

Menstruation

WINTER	CRONE	EARTH	DARK MOON

If you're not pregnant this cycle, you'll now be bleeding.

The day you start to bleed is day 1 of your cycle and this is the day to start charting. Depending on your cycle, your bleed can last anything from between three to eight or nine days and varies from person to person. The first few days of your cycle may leave you feeling achy and tired, but from day 3 onwards, your estrogen levels will start to rise again and you'll experience a boost in your energy, mood, optimism, and brain skills. When estrogen rises, it also boosts your levels of testosterone, and when this increases, it amps up your confidence, self-esteem and courage—but don't get too excited: on the days of your bleed, these happy hormones, while rising, are not high yet. In fact, in the first three or four days of your bleed, they are staying low so that you rest and immerse in self-care and preservation.

Now I know this isn't always easy—try to organize your life so that you can slow down a little in this phase.

So, you see, the rhythms of nature, the moon and our menstrual cycle provide us with our very own amazing inner teacher, guide, initiator and spiritual practice.

When you chart, you'll start to discover the best days to schedule a big meeting or to launch a business, and you'll understand why you argue with your partner on day 21 of your cycle *every* month.

Your cycle is your very own YOU-nique-to-you treasure map.

Hint: YOU are the treasure.

When you know this, life is better. You're more creative, you're more successful.

No self-help book has *ever* taught me that. Just saying.

Charting: The Details

So, from your next bleed, start to chart your cycle.

This is a practice; I recommend charting for *at least* three to six months so that you can really see the patterns and similarities and begin to start making sense of what you're charting. But, honestly? I've been doing it for *years* and I still learn something new about myself each and every cycle.

When to start? Day 1 of your menstrual cycle—and that's the first full day that you bleed.

Once you've marked down the date and declared it day 1, find out which phase the moon is in on day 1 of your bleed. To find this out, simply look up the date you begin bleeding on a lunar calendar— you can google "lunar calendar" to find out exactly what the moon's doing from one day to the next or download moon cycle apps like iLuna.

For example, if you start to bleed on January 4th, check the calendar to find out the phase of the moon. Record the date and the phases of both the moon and your menstrual cycle, and then chart your emotions, how you're feeling physically, mentally, spiritually, what you need, and then riff. Some days you'll have so much you want to say… and other days? Not so much.

What's great is when you start to recognize that those days when you have lots to say turn out to be around the same day of your cycle, every cycle. When you start to recognize patterns like this, you get to be a super-sleuth. Does this mean you have a lot to say, so you'd be super-chatty and could book time to be with friends? Or is it that these are days when you need to vent, and it's better that the vent stays in the pages of a journal and is not said out loud?

If you're moved to do so, you could also start charting the astrological journey as it, too, works on a cyclic basis. Throughout our entire 29-day moon and bleed cycle, the moon will pass through each of the astrological signs for around 2.5 days—so you might find that while you don't bleed exactly every 29 days, you might be bleeding every time the moon is in Virgo, for instance—seriously, the self-discovery is NEVER ENDING.

I LOVE it!

FYI: If this all feels wildly overwhelming and brand new, just know that you don't have to get it all right now. This is not meant to be "hard", it's a way of getting to know yourself, your tendencies, your needs, your superpowers—it's bloody incredible.

Cycle Scopes: Your Cycle at a Glance

To support your cycle-charting process, on the first day of your bleed—or if you're currently not bleeding but want to chart your moods and emotions along with the moon, on the day of the Dark Moon—work with and refer to these fun and informative cycle scopes to help you start to recognize what's ACTUALLY going on with your body and your cycle. Back in 2015, I created the #sharemycycle hashtag, where I shared my feels and my experience each day. At the time, I got lots of comments from people ick-ed out by it, but now, thankfully, that hashtag has been shared thousands of times, and social media is full of people talking about their bloody period and sharing their monthly menstrual experiences.

What I share here are super-short, sweet, and sometimes slightly tongue-in-cheek daily cycle scopes for a 28-ish day cycle. This is based on charting my own cycle and the cyclic energies that clients have shared with me. Please know that this may be absolutely NOT how it is for you.

I also know that many, many people don't have 28-day cycles, so I suggest letting these 28-day at-a-glance cycle "scopes" simply be a guide. Keep your own cycle journal so that you create your own cycle scopes that are specific to you, your body, and your own menstrual experience and wisdom.

Day 1: It's quite possible that on the first day of your bleed, your entire womb is falling out of your vagina, and you'll feel a combination of sore, sacred, and like you're feeling it ALL. Estrogen starts out at ground zero on day 1, so don't be surprised if from today through to day 3, you feel achy and tired—immerse yourself in self-care, radical rest, and preservation of the self-love kind.

Day 2: Rising estrogen and testosterone mean that you may feel the first signs of your energy and good vibes starting to return. Hurrah. Don't be fooled, though; while you may wake up feeling like you could do ALL. THE. THINGS, your body will most likely lose steam by mid-morning. Instead of blowing today's teeny bit of energy doing stuff that can be put off, take it sl-o-o-o-o-w. If you've got any big questions or decisions to make, bleed on it. Make a den, get comfy, place your hand on your womb, meditate, and heart riff. Let your womb be your oracle.

Day 3: As your estrogen and testosterone continue to rise, around day 3 you're able to start refocusing and wanting to make sense of the world, but don't be in too much of a rush to "get back out there." Your flow may still be heavy, and you may not be able to fully articulate what you actually want to say.

Day 4: I always find that day 4 marks the start of "fun" me. Energy levels are rising, a sense of optimism and confidence returns. I'm able to turn my attention to the outside world again. Your blood may start to change color and texture around day 4 too. If you experience a heavy flow, it may be showing signs of getting lighter.

Day 5: If you experience a "normal" flow (whatever one of *those* is), it should start to feel lighter, as should your mood. Today's the day to get creative—think up solutions to problems, make art, tackle the emails, start to explore any ideas and downloads you've received during the last few days.

Day 6: Today you think AND feel like Wonder Woman. That creativity you were experiencing yesterday? Forget it. Today you're all about the logic. Your estrogen and testosterone levels mean you have clarity and focus, and by now there's a chance you've also stopped bleeding too.

Day 7: The I-can-do-it-all vibes are HIGH, and you may notice a shift of energy as you move into the pre-ovulation phase. Tiny follicles on your ovaries are starting to form in preparation to release an egg, and while you're amped up and ready for anything, there's the potential for tiny dramas to turn into full-on anxiety-inducing stress-outs. You can blame estrogen for that.

Day 8: While you may be feeling practical, logical, and like a fully-functioning grown-up today, follicles are continuing to grow in preparation for the egg release, and the egg development is causing your estrogen levels to rise. That rising estrogen? It's why, despite the adulting, you're tempted to book a last-minute flight to LA, get a tattoo, and stay out dancing until 2 a.m..

Day 9: I like day 9 a LOT. It's my "I'm in control" day. Everything feels doable here, as if I might actually have got my shit together.

It's no surprise then that these hormones have us feeling like we've figured out adulting right at the same time that extra estrogen is thickening the lining of the uterus, getting it ready just in case an egg gets fertilized and needs a comfy place to grow for the next nine months. Our bodies are SMART.

Day 10: Ha! I laugh in the face of adulthood as estrogen is now sky-high *and* testosterone is rising toward its peak and has me wanting to take ALL the risks and say "Yes" to EVERYTHING.

Day 11: From now through until day 13, hormonally, you're on fire. THESE are the days to work late, to get shit done, make decisions, and DO. ALL. THE. THINGS. If you're looking to conceive, these are also the days to ramp up the amount of sex you're having too. Wink.

Day 12: Sound the sirens, this girl is on fiyaaaahhhhhhhhhh! If you thought yesterday was good, today just gets better. Energy levels and your ability to articulate are high; you're sharp, funny, and you're good to be around. This is the day I schedule any social events—it's a very small window of opportunity when this particularly introverted extrovert wants to "people".

Day 13: Today you're a total powerhouse: testosterone and estrogen are both now at their peak, you're fertile, and if it's what your body does, it will release an egg. You'll be feeling the potency. If you're not making out or making a baby, use this potent Creatrix power to create something else—a book, a project, or a piece of art.

Day 14: So testosterone and estrogen have peaked, and for some, day 14 is ovulation—but this isn't true for everyone. Check your vaginal fluid to be sure. If there's a lot of it, and if it's egg white-y in look and consistency, then there's a good chance you're ovulating. If you don't want to make a baby when your vag is producing the slippery stuff, you should deffo be using a barrier method, because THIS is the good stuff. When you're ovulating, you're magnetic, and your aura stretches to 26ft (that's an exaggeration, but y'know, it's big—use it).

Day 15: You'll still feel the good vibes from the last few days, but be prepared; as those hormone levels start to drop, so do your energy levels. The good news? Those energy levels don't drop right away, so if there's work to do, a project that you need concentration, focus, and brainpower for, use today's energetics to get it done. That egg? It's now journeying down the fallopian tube looking for some sperm action.

Day 16: Heads up, this is your last day to access the ability to concentrate, focus, and do all of that logical-brain thinking because, from here on in, you're going to start to wish you hadn't said "Yes" to "doing" quite so many things in the coming days. You'll feel less interested in socializing and more interested in having long baths filled with crystals, oils, and rose petals (wait, that might just be me?). Progesterone has entered and is encouraging you to become more self-nurturing and to choose comfy-ness over skydiving. Why? Because if there was sperm and egg action, it too will need nurturing and comfy-ness, NOT skydiving.

Day 17: So, today may feel like one big reality check. You see everything exactly as it is, and that's not always easy to do. Your uterus lining is thickening in case there's potential baby action, estrogen is dropping, while progesterone is high. Cue tears. ALL. THE TEARS. Or rage. Or both.

Day 18: Testosterone and estrogen appear to have changed their minds and start to rise again, but this time without all of the feel-good vibes they brought with them earlier in the cycle. Boo. Why? Because progesterone is basically a buzz-kill. Its job is to make sure that if an egg was fertilized in the last few days, your womb stays safe.

Day 19: Despite testosterone and estrogen rising, progesterone is still in charge. That's all.

Day 20: OK, so today, right through until you next bleed, trying to "make sense" of things starts to get a bit harder as you now move into emo, "all the feels" territory. If you're progesterone-sensitive, it may activate tears and confusion, and trying to do anything "practical" starts to get harder from here on in. I know, right? *Shakes fist at progesterone.*

Day 21: Between today and day 25, I'm not my most favorite person to be around. For these few days, I try not to schedule meetings or anything that involves people if I can possibly help it. In other news, the rising progesterone does make these few days good for clearing out, editing, and revising—it's the only day in my cycle you'll catch me with a hoover. Actual fact.

Day 22: Ohhh, today, progesterone peaks. This means that you may need at least one (preferably 84 in my case) nanna naps to overcome hormone-fuelled fatigue. I, for one, will not judge. Mainly because I'll be under my blanket napping too.

Day 23: ALL the hormones are now on the decrease. Of course they are. If you've any kind of big decision to make, put off making it until after you bleed, if you can. It's not that you can't trust yourself here, but this second half of the cycle is new territory for many of us, so until you're practiced at making emotional decisions with discernment, I recommend waiting until you return to day 6.

Day 24: Progesterone levels are still high in comparison to the rest of your hormones, which are plummeting about now. What does this mean? Well, for me, usually tears, rage, and chocolate. A lot of chocolate. Forever Cacao, my FAVORITE cacao supplier, is very well utilized between days 21 and 25.

Day 25: This has me showing up like Kali Ma incarnate: rage-full and angry, and without patience or tolerance. This is a tricky day for a lot of us as all the hormones are withdrawing at this point BUT, if channeled correctly—or if, in my case, I'm kept away from people—it can be a really creative time.

Day 26: Personally, I always feel a bit better after day 25, but lots of my clients feel those day-25 vibes waaay into day 26 too. I feel like if you KNOW the emotions that show up here (for example, rage is a big one for me), and you allow them, they can then move through a lot more easily. But if we're holding onto them, pushing them down, trying to ignore them, or worried we might explode, they can create pain. It's why our creativity is heightened here, so that we can make art/magic from the feels.

Day 27: Ohhh, thanks to those plummeting energy levels, everything may feel like it's in sl-o-o-o-o-o-w motion. You may be wanting to fight the many, many injustices in the world, but ultimately your energy levels make that a little difficult, so then you get frustrated, not just at your inability to be in action, but also at the state of the world, and so it goes. I often wake up wanting to eat ALL THE FOOD before 7 a.m. on day 27, so if you can make that food good and high in protein—not just family-size bags of chips—you'll thank me, I promise.

Day 28: If you can, stay away from social media, as your comparison and not-good-enough buttons can get REALLY pushed here, and the sharpness of your truth-telling tongue combined with the lack of brainpower to articulate totally effectively makes social media a not-so-great space to be. If you're not pregnant, there's a good chance that your period is on its way.

Tracking and working with your cycle isn't a prescription for how to be and act on each and every day. (I mean, it can be, but would you really want it to be?) Instead, see it as a way to explore and get curious about your body. Learn what it's up to and understand how, based on your cyclic self-knowledge, you can let it provide you with insight and wisdom as to why you feel like you do and how you "could" show up.

How to Use Your Journal

Your *Red Journal* has 13 cycles for you to fill with all your cyclic intel.

Make this as practical or creative as feels good to you. It's your journal, it's your cyclic intel.

You'll find that there's space for you to chart what day and phase of the menstrual month you're currently in, what phase the moon is in and what astrological and planetary actions are at play too.

There's also an opportunity to journal.

So what exactly are you journaling?

Again, this is totally up to you, but here's what I'd recommend:

A 'down there' daily analysis

Tracking your menstrual health and wellness by knowing what's going on "down there":

- Am I dry?

- Am I juicy?

- Am I bleeding?

Feeling the feelings

A daily check in on the more dominant feelings and sensations.

- Your energy level

- Your mood

- Your dreams
- Your relationship to others
- Your sex drive

Self-sourcing

Curate and create a personal-to-you self-sourcing practice based on what you're experiencing.

- What movement have you done? What movement would feel good?
- Where's your head at?
- Where have you experienced pleasure? What would you need today for pleasure to occur?
- What have you done to nourish yourself? What would feel good that you haven't done already?

What's self-sourcing?

I've been sharing how to self-source with people for a few years now, and as with everything I share, it's *not* a formula, it's a process of self-discovery and exploration. Look, you do not need me to tell you to drink water, move your body and eat less sugar—I am not your mumma (also there's a ton of books and reading material online if that's the kind of information you're looking for). Self-sourcing is an invitation, through tracking, to get curious.

Cyclical wisdom is the foundation of how I self-source. I work with the phases of my menstrual cycle and the cycles of the moon to explore this.

Working with the ebb and flow of these cycles and the changing phases allows you to connect to your ever-changing cyclical inner landscape—your emotional, physical, and mental landscape—so that you can recognize what you need in order to feel resourced and vital and fully alive in each phase.

When I first charted, I recognized I needed different exercise practices for each phase—I like to jog and get sweaty in my pre-ovulation and ovulation phases and like to do very little in premenstruation and menstruation. Ha! I prefer different sexual positions in different phases, my food and taste preferences are different in each phase, and, because of my heightened sensorial nature in the premenstrual phase, I can be absolutely repulsed by a perfume in that phase that I love in pre-ovulation. So chart it alllllll and you'll quickly begin to recognize what you need to tend to and how to support yourself in each phase.

Self-reflection

At the end of each cycle you'll find space for self-reflection.
This is my favorite bit.

This is where you get to turn super-sleuth on yourself and pick up clues and cues as to what is *actually* going on in your body from cycle to cycle.

- Which cycle days were most positive?

- Which were most challenging?

- What patterns are unfolding?

This is where you can leave notes for your next-cycle self. This is so bloody useful. One of the big things that kept coming up for me is: "Stop saying yes to things on day 11 and 12 (my pre-ovulation phase, when everything feels totally possible and doable) that you know you won't want to actually do on day 23 (my premenstrual phase, when I am not good at—or honestly interested in—people-ing). In *Code Red*, I mention that, through charting, I learnt very quickly for my benefit, and that of my hot Viking husband, that day 25 was a day when I needed to NOT be around people or on social media. I'm rage-full, should only be spoken to if it's an emergency, and even then, make sure you approach with caution. And chocolate.

Make the process of charting and tracking your own

Some people love to go full Creatrix and pick a color to represent each phase of the cycle, and use symbols, diagrams, and stickers to illustrate moods and sensations. Others really love the opportunity to journal and heart riff on what's coming up for them each day, while others simply want to fill in the chart that you'll find at the beginning of each cycle by picking one word to sum up their cyclic experience for that day.

Obviously, I like to do it ALL. Ha!

I love any excuse to get creative with color and stickers. I like to have the option for a quick, at-a-glance overview of that month's cyclic experience and I like to journal what I'm feeling and experiencing every day because it helps me to track, connect to, and find ways to support the entire experience of how it is to be me.

My hope is that you make your *Red Journal* your own, that you carry it with you daily, make the act of filling it a fun and playful experience, and that in the process you discover lots of insight and wisdom about yourself that helps, supports, and guides you as you navigate your inner and outer landscape.

Your Daily Journal Entry

I'm pretty sure you don't need me to tell you how to use a journal, but simply use the headings I've shared here as a guide to fill in your findings as you explore your menstrual experience.

Here's an extract from one of my *Red Journal* entries...

Date: *22/05/2020*   Cycle day: *12*
Cycle phase: *Pre-ovulation*   Moon phase: *New*
Day/planetary energy: *Wednesday, Mercury*   Sun sign: *Gemini*

The Feels

Slept well – 7.5 hours, very talkative (which is unlike me) energy levels high and feeling particularly minxy today. Wink.

Self-sourcing

Danced to 20 minutes of "90s boybands" playlist, wore a red lip and had an art date in nature with myself so that I didn't stay at my desk all day.

Heart Riffs

This is the third cycle where, on day 12, I've felt super-chatty so I'm making a note to schedule clients and phone convos for this day every cycle.

Your Monthly Cycle Wheel

Fill in your cycle wheel as a quick one-word reference for those days when you might be too busy to fill in the journal pages right away, or use it as a touchpoint to oversee your whole cycle.

Here's one of my filled-in cycle wheels for you to use as a guide.

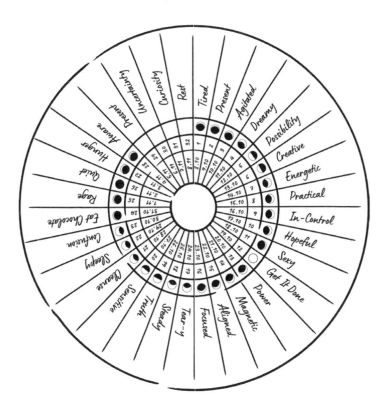

Your Journal

Your Cycle Wheel

Start date: 1/2

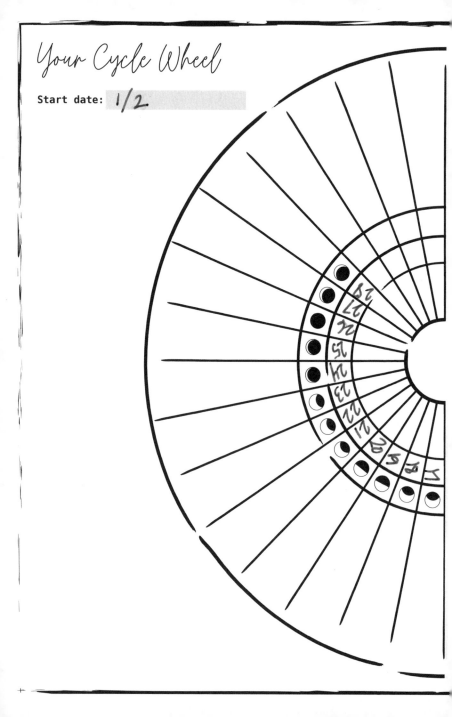

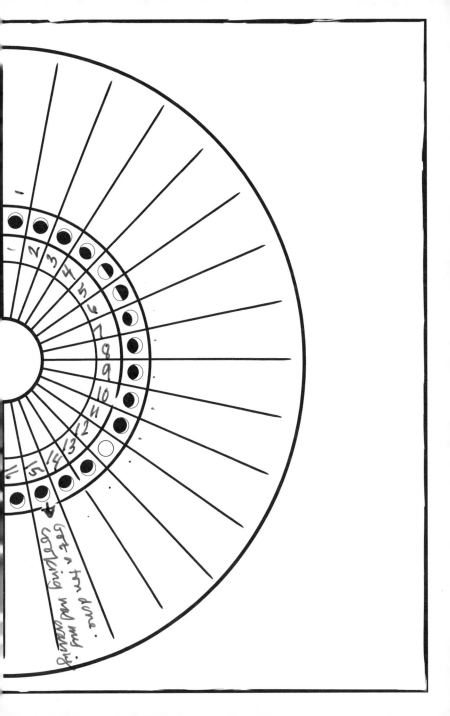

Date: Cycle day:

Cycle phase: Moon phase:

Day/planetary energy: Sun sign:

The Feels

Self-sourcing

Heart Riffs

Date: Cycle day:

Cycle phase: Moon phase:

Day/planetary energy: Sun sign:

The Feels

Self-sourcing

Heart Riffs

Date: Cycle day:

Cycle phase: Moon phase:

Day/planetary energy: Sun sign:

The Feels

_____

_____

_____

Self-sourcing

_____

_____

_____

Heart Riffs

_____

_____

_____

_____

Date: Cycle day:

Cycle phase: Moon phase:

Day/planetary energy: Sun sign:

The Feels

_____

_____

_____

Self-sourcing

_____

_____

_____

Heart Riffs

_____

_____

_____

_____

Date: Cycle day:

Cycle phase: Moon phase:

Day/planetary energy: Sun sign:

The Feels 🤲

_____

_____

_____

Self-sourcing 🧘

_____

_____

_____

Heart Riffs ✍️

_____

_____

_____

_____

Date: Cycle day:

Cycle phase: Moon phase:

Day/planetary energy: Sun sign:

The Feels 🤲

_____

_____

_____

Self-sourcing 🧘

_____

_____

_____

Heart Riffs ✍️

_____

_____

_____

_____

Date: Cycle day:

Cycle phase: Moon phase:

Day/planetary energy: Sun sign:

The Feels

Self-sourcing

Heart Riffs

Date: Cycle day:

Cycle phase: Moon phase:

Day/planetary energy: Sun sign:

The Feels

Self-sourcing

Heart Riffs

Date: _____ Cycle day: _____

Cycle phase: _____ Moon phase: _____

Day/planetary energy: _____ Sun sign: _____

The Feels ✋

_____

_____

_____

Self-sourcing 🧘

_____

_____

_____

Heart Riffs ✍

_____

_____

_____

_____

Date: _____ Cycle day: _____

Cycle phase: _____ Moon phase: _____

Day/planetary energy: _____ Sun sign: _____

The Feels ✋

_____

_____

_____

Self-sourcing 🧘

_____

_____

_____

Heart Riffs ✍

_____

_____

_____

_____

Date: _____ Cycle day: _____
Cycle phase: _____ Moon phase: _____
Day/planetary energy: _____ Sun sign: _____

The Feels 🫶

_____
_____
_____
_____

Self-sourcing 🧘

_____
_____
_____
_____

Heart Riffs ✍️

_____
_____
_____
_____

Date: _____ Cycle day: _____
Cycle phase: _____ Moon phase: _____
Day/planetary energy: _____ Sun sign: _____

The Feels 🫶

_____
_____
_____
_____

Self-sourcing 🧘

_____
_____
_____
_____

Heart Riffs ✍️

_____
_____
_____
_____

Date: _____ Cycle day: _____
Cycle phase: _____ Moon phase: _____
Day/planetary energy: _____ Sun sign: _____

The Feels 🤲

_____
_____
_____
_____

Self-sourcing 🧘

_____
_____
_____
_____

Heart Riffs ✍️

_____
_____
_____
_____

Date: _____ Cycle day: _____
Cycle phase: _____ Moon phase: _____
Day/planetary energy: _____ Sun sign: _____

The Feels 🤲

_____
_____
_____
_____

Self-sourcing 🧘

_____
_____
_____
_____

Heart Riffs ✍️

_____
_____
_____
_____

Date: Cycle day:

Cycle phase: Moon phase:

Day/planetary energy: Sun sign:

The Feels

_____

_____

_____

_____

Self-sourcing

_____

_____

_____

Heart Riffs

_____

_____

_____

_____

Date: Cycle day:

Cycle phase: Moon phase:

Day/planetary energy: Sun sign:

The Feels

_____

_____

_____

_____

Self-sourcing

_____

_____

_____

Heart Riffs

_____

_____

_____

_____

Date: _____ Cycle day: _____

Cycle phase: _____ Moon phase: _____

Day/planetary energy: _____ Sun sign: _____

The Feels 🫶

_____

_____

_____

_____

Self-sourcing 🧘

_____

_____

_____

_____

Heart Riffs ✍️

_____

_____

_____

_____

Date: _____ Cycle day: _____

Cycle phase: _____ Moon phase: _____

Day/planetary energy: _____ Sun sign: _____

The Feels 🫶

_____

_____

_____

_____

Self-sourcing 🧘

_____

_____

_____

_____

Heart Riffs ✍️

_____

_____

_____

_____

Date: _____   Cycle day: _____
Cycle phase: _____   Moon phase: _____
Day/planetary energy: _____   Sun sign: _____

The Feels 🫶

_____
_____
_____
_____

Self-sourcing 🧘

_____
_____
_____
_____

Heart Riffs ✍️

_____
_____
_____
_____

Date: _____   Cycle day: _____
Cycle phase: _____   Moon phase: _____
Day/planetary energy: _____   Sun sign: _____

The Feels 🫶

_____
_____
_____
_____

Self-sourcing 🧘

_____
_____
_____
_____

Heart Riffs ✍️

_____
_____
_____
_____

Date: _____ Cycle day: _____
Cycle phase: _____ Moon phase: _____
Day/planetary energy: _____ Sun sign: _____

The Feels 🫶

_____
_____
_____
_____

Self-sourcing 🧘

_____
_____
_____
_____

Heart Riffs ✍️

_____
_____
_____
_____

Date: _____ Cycle day: _____
Cycle phase: _____ Moon phase: _____
Day/planetary energy: _____ Sun sign: _____

The Feels 🫶

_____
_____
_____
_____

Self-sourcing 🧘

_____
_____
_____
_____

Heart Riffs ✍️

_____
_____
_____
_____

Date: Cycle day:

Cycle phase: Moon phase:

Day/planetary energy: Sun sign:

The Feels ✋

_____

_____

_____

_____

Self-sourcing 🧘

_____

_____

_____

Heart Riffs ✍

_____

_____

_____

_____

Date: Cycle day:

Cycle phase: Moon phase:

Day/planetary energy: Sun sign:

The Feels ✋

_____

_____

_____

_____

Self-sourcing 🧘

_____

_____

_____

Heart Riffs ✍

_____

_____

_____

_____

Date: Cycle day:

Cycle phase: Moon phase:

Day/planetary energy: Sun sign:

The Feels

_____

_____

_____

_____

Self-sourcing

_____

_____

_____

Heart Riffs

_____

_____

_____

_____

Date: Cycle day:

Cycle phase: Moon phase:

Day/planetary energy: Sun sign:

The Feels

_____

_____

_____

_____

Self-sourcing

_____

_____

_____

Heart Riffs

_____

_____

_____

_____

Date: _____   Cycle day: _____
Cycle phase: _____   Moon phase: _____
Day/planetary energy: _____   Sun sign: _____

The Feels 🖐️

_____
_____
_____
_____

Self-sourcing 🧘

_____
_____
_____

Heart Riffs ✍️

_____
_____
_____
_____

Date: _____   Cycle day: _____
Cycle phase: _____   Moon phase: _____
Day/planetary energy: _____   Sun sign: _____

The Feels 🖐️

_____
_____
_____
_____

Self-sourcing 🧘

_____
_____
_____

Heart Riffs ✍️

_____
_____
_____
_____

Date: Cycle day:
Cycle phase: Moon phase:
Day/planetary energy: Sun sign:

The Feels ✋

_____
_____
_____
_____

Self-sourcing 🧘

_____
_____
_____
_____

Heart Riffs ✍

_____
_____
_____
_____

Date: 1/16/21   Cycle day: 16
Cycle phase: Moon phase:
Day/planetary energy: Sun sign:

The Feels ✋

In control, in the zone, easy to
laugh + indulge. Sexy. Open.

Self-sourcing 🧘

Cook! De-clutter! These felt
awesome.

Heart Riffs ✍

_____
_____
_____
_____

Date: 1/17/21   Cycle day: 16
Cycle phase: Moon phase:
Day/planetary energy: Sun sign:

The Feels 🫶

_____
_____
_____
_____

Self-sourcing 🧘

_____
_____
_____
_____

Heart Riffs ✍️

_____
_____
_____
_____
_____

Date: Cycle day:
Cycle phase: Moon phase:
Day/planetary energy: Sun sign:

The Feels 🫶

_____
_____
_____
_____

Self-sourcing 🧘

_____
_____
_____
_____

Heart Riffs ✍️

_____
_____
_____
_____
_____

Reflect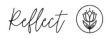

Which cycle days were most positive?

_____

_____

_____

_____

_____

_____

_____

Which were most challenging?

_____

_____

_____

_____

_____

_____

_____

_____

_____

What patterns are unfolding?

Notes for your next-cycle self…

Your Cycle Wheel

Start date:

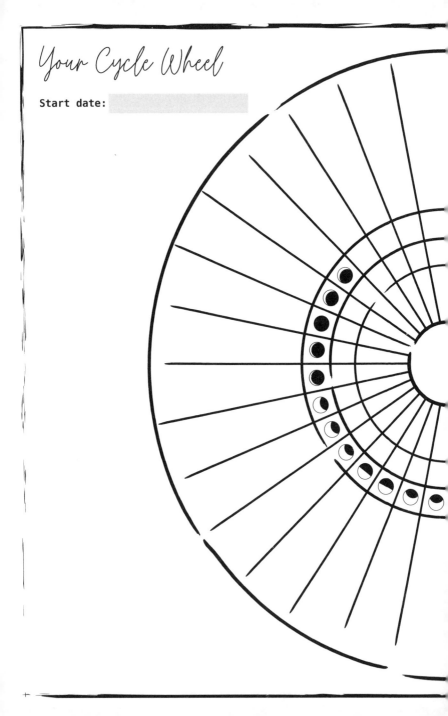

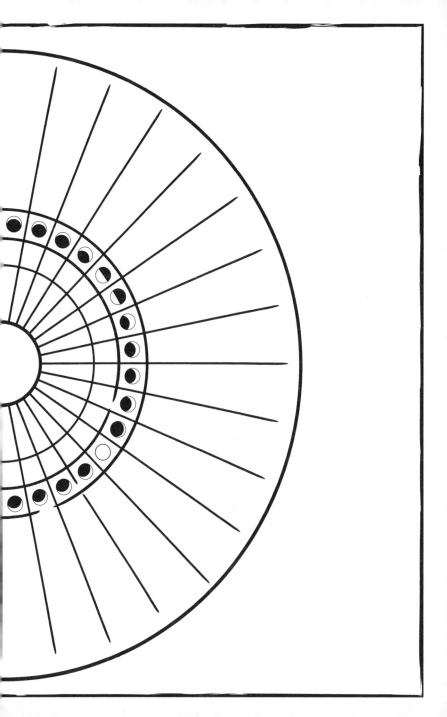

Date: ‗‗‗‗‗‗‗‗‗ Cycle day: ‗‗‗‗‗‗‗

Cycle phase: ‗‗‗‗‗‗‗ Moon phase: ‗‗‗‗‗‗‗‗

Day/planetary energy: ‗‗‗‗‗‗‗ Sun sign: ‗‗‗‗‗‗

The Feels 🫶

‗‗‗
‗‗‗
‗‗‗
‗‗‗

Self-sourcing 🧘

‗‗‗
‗‗‗
‗‗‗
‗‗‗

Heart Riffs ✍️

‗‗‗
‗‗‗
‗‗‗
‗‗‗

Date: ‗‗‗‗‗‗‗‗‗ Cycle day: ‗‗‗‗‗‗‗

Cycle phase: ‗‗‗‗‗‗‗ Moon phase: ‗‗‗‗‗‗‗‗

Day/planetary energy: ‗‗‗‗‗‗‗ Sun sign: ‗‗‗‗‗‗

The Feels 🫶

‗‗‗
‗‗‗
‗‗‗
‗‗‗

Self-sourcing 🧘

‗‗‗
‗‗‗
‗‗‗
‗‗‗

Heart Riffs ✍️

‗‗‗
‗‗‗
‗‗‗
‗‗‗

Date: [blank] Cycle day: [blank]

Cycle phase: [blank] Moon phase: [blank]

Day/planetary energy: [blank] Sun sign: [blank]

The Feels

_____

_____

_____

Self-sourcing

_____

_____

_____

Heart Riffs

_____

_____

_____

_____

Date: [blank] Cycle day: [blank]

Cycle phase: [blank] Moon phase: [blank]

Day/planetary energy: [blank] Sun sign: [blank]

The Feels

_____

_____

_____

Self-sourcing

_____

_____

_____

Heart Riffs

_____

_____

_____

Date: _____ Cycle day: _____

Cycle phase: _____ Moon phase: _____

Day/planetary energy: _____ Sun sign: _____

The Feels 🫱

_____

_____

_____

Self-sourcing 🧘

_____

_____

_____

Heart Riffs ✍️

_____

_____

_____

_____

Date: _____ Cycle day: _____

Cycle phase: _____ Moon phase: _____

Day/planetary energy: _____ Sun sign: _____

The Feels 🫱

_____

_____

_____

Self-sourcing 🧘

_____

_____

_____

Heart Riffs ✍️

_____

_____

_____

_____

Date: _____ Cycle day: _____

Cycle phase: _____ Moon phase: _____

Day/planetary energy: _____ Sun sign: _____

The Feels ✋

_____

_____

_____

_____

Self-sourcing 🧘

_____

_____

_____

Heart Riffs ✍️

_____

_____

_____

_____

Date: _____ Cycle day: _____

Cycle phase: _____ Moon phase: _____

Day/planetary energy: _____ Sun sign: _____

The Feels ✋

_____

_____

_____

_____

Self-sourcing 🧘

_____

_____

_____

Heart Riffs ✍️

_____

_____

_____

_____

Date: Cycle day:

Cycle phase: Moon phase:

Day/planetary energy: Sun sign:

The Feels

Self-sourcing

Heart Riffs

Date: Cycle day:

Cycle phase: Moon phase:

Day/planetary energy: Sun sign:

The Feels

Self-sourcing

Heart Riffs

Date: _____ Cycle day: _____
Cycle phase: _____ Moon phase: _____
Day/planetary energy: _____ Sun sign: _____

The Feels ✋

_____
_____
_____
_____

Self-sourcing 🧘

_____
_____
_____

Heart Riffs ✍

_____
_____
_____
_____

Date: _____ Cycle day: _____
Cycle phase: _____ Moon phase: _____
Day/planetary energy: _____ Sun sign: _____

The Feels ✋

_____
_____
_____
_____

Self-sourcing 🧘

_____
_____
_____

Heart Riffs ✍

_____
_____
_____
_____

Date: _____ Cycle day: _____

Cycle phase: _____ Moon phase: _____

Day/planetary energy: _____ Sun sign: _____

The Feels 🤲

_____

_____

_____

_____

Self-sourcing 🧘

_____

_____

_____

_____

Heart Riffs ✍️

_____

_____

_____

_____

Date: _____ Cycle day: _____

Cycle phase: _____ Moon phase: _____

Day/planetary energy: _____ Sun sign: _____

The Feels 🤲

_____

_____

_____

_____

Self-sourcing 🧘

_____

_____

_____

_____

Heart Riffs ✍️

_____

_____

_____

_____

Date: Cycle day:

Cycle phase: Moon phase:

Day/planetary energy: Sun sign:

The Feels

Self-sourcing

Heart Riffs

Date: Cycle day:

Cycle phase: Moon phase:

Day/planetary energy: Sun sign:

The Feels

Self-sourcing

Heart Riffs

Date: Cycle day:

Cycle phase: Moon phase:

Day/planetary energy: Sun sign:

The Feels ✋

Self-sourcing 🧘

Heart Riffs ✍️

Date: Cycle day:

Cycle phase: Moon phase:

Day/planetary energy: Sun sign:

The Feels ✋

Self-sourcing 🧘

Heart Riffs ✍️

Date: _____ Cycle day: _____

Cycle phase: _____ Moon phase: _____

Day/planetary energy: _____ Sun sign: _____

The Feels 🫶

_____

_____

_____

Self-sourcing 🧘

_____

_____

_____

Heart Riffs ✍️

_____

_____

_____

_____

Date: _____ Cycle day: _____

Cycle phase: _____ Moon phase: _____

Day/planetary energy: _____ Sun sign: _____

The Feels 🫶

_____

_____

_____

Self-sourcing 🧘

_____

_____

_____

Heart Riffs ✍️

_____

_____

_____

_____

Date: _____   Cycle day: _____
Cycle phase: _____   Moon phase: _____
Day/planetary energy: _____   Sun sign: _____

The Feels ✋

_____
_____
_____
_____

Self-sourcing 🧘

_____
_____
_____
_____

Heart Riffs ✍

_____
_____
_____
_____

Date: _____   Cycle day: _____
Cycle phase: _____   Moon phase: _____
Day/planetary energy: _____   Sun sign: _____

The Feels ✋

_____
_____
_____
_____

Self-sourcing 🧘

_____
_____
_____
_____

Heart Riffs ✍

_____
_____
_____
_____

Date: _____ Cycle day: _____
Cycle phase: _____ Moon phase: _____
Day/planetary energy: _____ Sun sign: _____

The Feels ✍

_____
_____
_____

Self-sourcing 🧘

_____
_____
_____

Heart Riffs ✍

_____
_____
_____
_____

Date: _____ Cycle day: _____
Cycle phase: _____ Moon phase: _____
Day/planetary energy: _____ Sun sign: _____

The Feels ✍

_____
_____
_____

Self-sourcing 🧘

_____
_____
_____

Heart Riffs ✍

_____
_____
_____

Date: Cycle day:

Cycle phase: Moon phase:

Day/planetary energy: Sun sign:

The Feels

_____
_____
_____
_____

Self-sourcing

_____
_____
_____
_____

Heart Riffs

_____
_____
_____
_____

Date: Cycle day:

Cycle phase: Moon phase:

Day/planetary energy: Sun sign:

The Feels

_____
_____
_____
_____

Self-sourcing

_____
_____
_____
_____

Heart Riffs

_____
_____
_____
_____

Date: _____ Cycle day: _____

Cycle phase: _____ Moon phase: _____

Day/planetary energy: _____ Sun sign: _____

The Feels 🤲

_____

_____

_____

Self-sourcing 🧘

_____

_____

_____

Heart Riffs ✍️

_____

_____

_____

Date: _____ Cycle day: _____

Cycle phase: _____ Moon phase: _____

Day/planetary energy: _____ Sun sign: _____

The Feels 🤲

_____

_____

_____

Self-sourcing 🧘

_____

_____

_____

Heart Riffs ✍️

_____

_____

_____

Date: _____ Cycle day: _____

Cycle phase: _____ Moon phase: _____

Day/planetary energy: _____ Sun sign: _____

The Feels ✋

_____

_____

_____

Self-sourcing 🧘

_____

_____

_____

Heart Riffs ✍

_____

_____

_____

_____

Date: _____ Cycle day: _____

Cycle phase: _____ Moon phase: _____

Day/planetary energy: _____ Sun sign: _____

The Feels ✋

_____

_____

_____

Self-sourcing 🧘

_____

_____

_____

Heart Riffs ✍

_____

_____

_____

_____

Date: _____ Cycle day: _____

Cycle phase: _____ Moon phase: _____

Day/planetary energy: _____ Sun sign: _____

The Feels 🫶

_____

_____

_____

Self-sourcing 🧘

_____

_____

_____

Heart Riffs ✍️

_____

_____

_____

_____

Date: _____ Cycle day: _____

Cycle phase: _____ Moon phase: _____

Day/planetary energy: _____ Sun sign: _____

The Feels 🫶

_____

_____

_____

Self-sourcing 🧘

_____

_____

_____

Heart Riffs ✍️

_____

_____

_____

_____

Reflect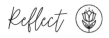

Which cycle days were most positive?

....

....

....

....

....

....

....

Which were most challenging?

....

....

....

....

....

....

....

....

What patterns are unfolding?

....

....

....

....

....

....

....

....

Notes for your next-cycle self...

....

....

....

....

....

....

....

....

....

Your Cycle Wheel

Start date:

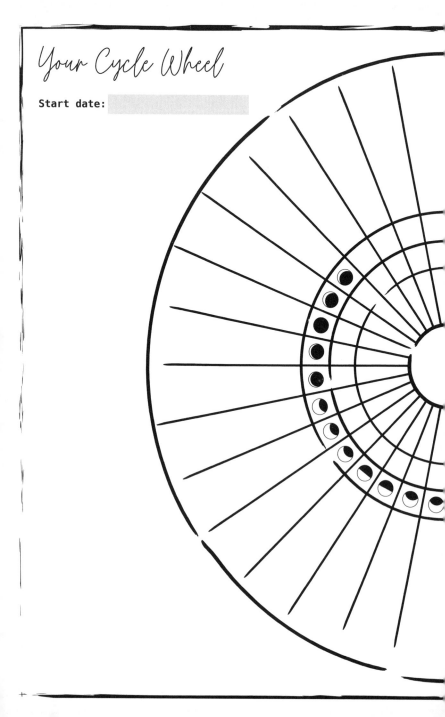

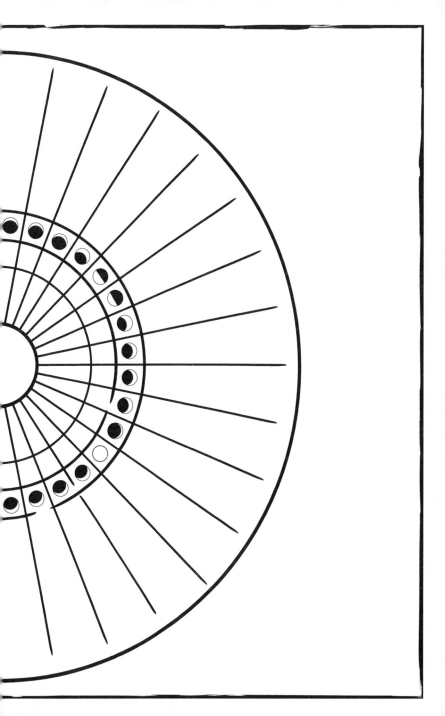

Date: _____ Cycle day: _____

Cycle phase: _____ Moon phase: _____

Day/planetary energy: _____ Sun sign: _____

The Feels 🫶

_____

_____

_____

Self-sourcing 🧘

_____

_____

_____

Heart Riffs ✍️

_____

_____

_____

_____

Date: _____ Cycle day: _____

Cycle phase: _____ Moon phase: _____

Day/planetary energy: _____ Sun sign: _____

The Feels 🫶

_____

_____

_____

Self-sourcing 🧘

_____

_____

_____

Heart Riffs ✍️

_____

_____

_____

Date: _____ Cycle day: _____

Cycle phase: _____ Moon phase: _____

Day/planetary energy: _____ Sun sign: _____

The Feels 🤲

_____

_____

_____

_____

Self-sourcing 🧘

_____

_____

_____

_____

Heart Riffs ✍️

_____

_____

_____

_____

Date: _____ Cycle day: _____

Cycle phase: _____ Moon phase: _____

Day/planetary energy: _____ Sun sign: _____

The Feels 🤲

_____

_____

_____

_____

Self-sourcing 🧘

_____

_____

_____

_____

Heart Riffs ✍️

_____

_____

_____

_____

Date: Cycle day:

Cycle phase: Moon phase:

Day/planetary energy: Sun sign:

The Feels

Self-sourcing

Heart Riffs

Date: Cycle day:

Cycle phase: Moon phase:

Day/planetary energy: Sun sign:

The Feels

Self-sourcing

Heart Riffs

Date: _____ Cycle day: _____

Cycle phase: _____ Moon phase: _____

Day/planetary energy: _____ Sun sign: _____

The Feels 🤟

_____

_____

_____

Self-sourcing 🧘

_____

_____

_____

Heart Riffs ✍️

_____

_____

_____

_____

Date: _____ Cycle day: _____

Cycle phase: _____ Moon phase: _____

Day/planetary energy: _____ Sun sign: _____

The Feels 🤟

_____

_____

_____

Self-sourcing 🧘

_____

_____

_____

Heart Riffs ✍️

_____

_____

_____

_____

Date: Cycle day:
Cycle phase: Moon phase:
Day/planetary energy: Sun sign:

The Feels 🫶

_____
_____
_____
_____

Self-sourcing 🧘

_____
_____
_____
_____

Heart Riffs ✍️

_____
_____
_____
_____

Date: Cycle day:
Cycle phase: Moon phase:
Day/planetary energy: Sun sign:

The Feels 🫶

_____
_____
_____
_____

Self-sourcing 🧘

_____
_____
_____
_____

Heart Riffs ✍️

_____
_____
_____
_____

Date: _____ Cycle day: _____
Cycle phase: _____ Moon phase: _____
Day/planetary energy: _____ Sun sign: _____

The Feels 🫶

_____
_____
_____
_____

Self-sourcing 🧘

_____
_____
_____
_____

Heart Riffs ✍️

_____
_____
_____
_____

Date: _____ Cycle day: _____
Cycle phase: _____ Moon phase: _____
Day/planetary energy: _____ Sun sign: _____

The Feels 🫶

_____
_____
_____
_____

Self-sourcing 🧘

_____
_____
_____
_____

Heart Riffs ✍️

_____
_____
_____
_____

Date: _____ Cycle day: _____

Cycle phase: _____ Moon phase: _____

Day/planetary energy: _____ Sun sign: _____

The Feels 🫶

_____

_____

_____

_____

Self-sourcing 🧘

_____

_____

_____

_____

Heart Riffs ✍️

_____

_____

_____

_____

Date: _____ Cycle day: _____

Cycle phase: _____ Moon phase: _____

Day/planetary energy: _____ Sun sign: _____

The Feels 🫶

_____

_____

_____

_____

Self-sourcing 🧘

_____

_____

_____

_____

Heart Riffs ✍️

_____

_____

_____

_____

Date: [blank]   Cycle day: [blank]
Cycle phase: [blank]   Moon phase: [blank]
Day/planetary energy: [blank]   Sun sign: [blank]

The Feels 🫶

_____
_____
_____
_____

Self-sourcing 🧘

_____
_____
_____
_____

Heart Riffs ✍️

_____
_____
_____
_____

Date: [blank]   Cycle day: [blank]
Cycle phase: [blank]   Moon phase: [blank]
Day/planetary energy: [blank]   Sun sign: [blank]

The Feels 🫶

_____
_____
_____
_____

Self-sourcing 🧘

_____
_____
_____
_____

Heart Riffs ✍️

_____
_____
_____
_____

Date: _____ Cycle day: _____

Cycle phase: _____ Moon phase: _____

Day/planetary energy: _____ Sun sign: _____

The Feels

_____

_____

_____

Self-sourcing

_____

_____

_____

Heart Riffs

_____

_____

_____

_____

Date: _____ Cycle day: _____

Cycle phase: _____ Moon phase: _____

Day/planetary energy: _____ Sun sign: _____

The Feels

_____

_____

_____

Self-sourcing

_____

_____

_____

Heart Riffs

_____

_____

_____

_____

Date: _____ Cycle day: _____

Cycle phase: _____ Moon phase: _____

Day/planetary energy: _____ Sun sign: _____

The Feels 🫶

_____

_____

_____

Self-sourcing 🧘

_____

_____

_____

Heart Riffs ✍️

_____

_____

_____

_____

Date: _____ Cycle day: _____

Cycle phase: _____ Moon phase: _____

Day/planetary energy: _____ Sun sign: _____

The Feels 🫶

_____

_____

_____

Self-sourcing 🧘

_____

_____

_____

Heart Riffs ✍️

_____

_____

_____

Date: _____ Cycle day: _____

Cycle phase: _____ Moon phase: _____

Day/planetary energy: _____ Sun sign: _____

The Feels 🫶

_____

_____

_____

Self-sourcing 🧘

_____

_____

_____

Heart Riffs ✍️

_____

_____

_____

_____

Date: _____ Cycle day: _____

Cycle phase: _____ Moon phase: _____

Day/planetary energy: _____ Sun sign: _____

The Feels 🫶

_____

_____

_____

Self-sourcing 🧘

_____

_____

_____

Heart Riffs ✍️

_____

_____

_____

_____

Date: _____ Cycle day: _____
Cycle phase: _____ Moon phase: _____
Day/planetary energy: _____ Sun sign: _____

The Feels 🤲

_____
_____
_____
_____

Self-sourcing 🧘

_____
_____
_____
_____

Heart Riffs ✍️

_____
_____
_____
_____

Date: _____ Cycle day: _____
Cycle phase: _____ Moon phase: _____
Day/planetary energy: _____ Sun sign: _____

The Feels 🤲

_____
_____
_____
_____

Self-sourcing 🧘

_____
_____
_____
_____

Heart Riffs ✍️

_____
_____
_____
_____

Date: _____ Cycle day: _____

Cycle phase: _____ Moon phase: _____

Day/planetary energy: _____ Sun sign: _____

The Feels 🫶

_____

_____

_____

_____

Self-sourcing 🧘

_____

_____

_____

Heart Riffs ✍️

_____

_____

_____

_____

Date: _____ Cycle day: _____

Cycle phase: _____ Moon phase: _____

Day/planetary energy: _____ Sun sign: _____

The Feels 🫶

_____

_____

_____

_____

Self-sourcing 🧘

_____

_____

_____

Heart Riffs ✍️

_____

_____

_____

_____

Date: _____ Cycle day: _____

Cycle phase: _____ Moon phase: _____

Day/planetary energy: _____ Sun sign: _____

The Feels 🤲

_____

_____

_____

_____

Self-sourcing 🧘

_____

_____

_____

_____

Heart Riffs ✍️

_____

_____

_____

_____

Date: _____ Cycle day: _____

Cycle phase: _____ Moon phase: _____

Day/planetary energy: _____ Sun sign: _____

The Feels 🤲

_____

_____

_____

_____

Self-sourcing 🧘

_____

_____

_____

_____

Heart Riffs ✍️

_____

_____

_____

_____

Date: Cycle day:
Cycle phase: Moon phase:
Day/planetary energy: Sun sign:

The Feels ✍

_____
_____
_____
_____

Self-sourcing 🧘

_____
_____
_____

Heart Riffs ✍

_____
_____
_____
_____

Date: Cycle day:
Cycle phase: Moon phase:
Day/planetary energy: Sun sign:

The Feels ✍

_____
_____
_____
_____

Self-sourcing 🧘

_____
_____
_____

Heart Riffs ✍

_____
_____
_____
_____

Date: _____ Cycle day: _____

Cycle phase: _____ Moon phase: _____

Day/planetary energy: _____ Sun sign: _____

The Feels ✋

_____

_____

_____

_____

Self-sourcing 🧘

_____

_____

_____

Heart Riffs ✍

_____

_____

_____

_____

Date: _____ Cycle day: _____

Cycle phase: _____ Moon phase: _____

Day/planetary energy: _____ Sun sign: _____

The Feels ✋

_____

_____

_____

_____

Self-sourcing 🧘

_____

_____

_____

Heart Riffs ✍

_____

_____

_____

_____

Reflect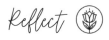

Which cycle days were most positive?

_____

_____

_____

_____

_____

_____

_____

_____

Which were most challenging?

_____

_____

_____

_____

_____

_____

_____

_____

_____

What patterns are unfolding?

....

....

....

....

....

....

....

Notes for your next-cycle self…

....

....

....

....

....

....

....

....

Your Cycle Wheel

Start date:

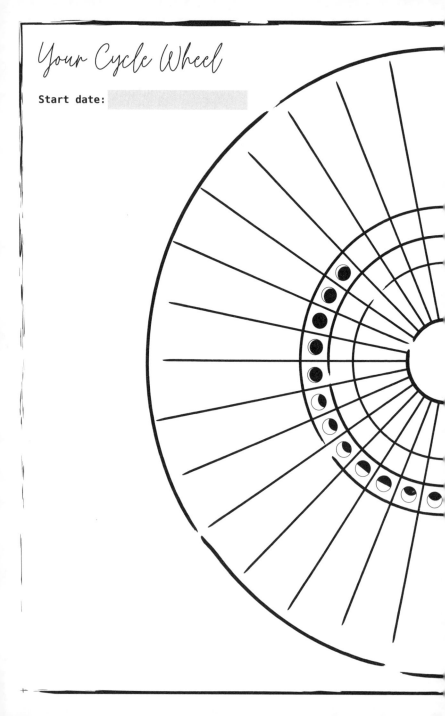

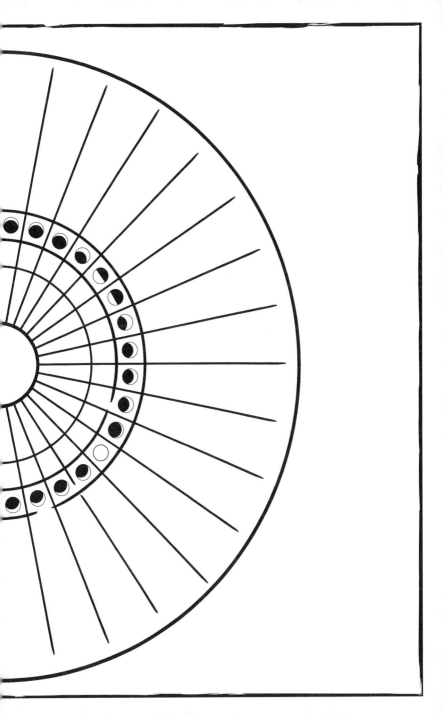

Date: Cycle day:

Cycle phase: Moon phase:

Day/planetary energy: Sun sign:

The Feels

Self-sourcing

Heart Riffs

Date: Cycle day:

Cycle phase: Moon phase:

Day/planetary energy: Sun sign:

The Feels

Self-sourcing

Heart Riffs

Date: _____ Cycle day: _____

Cycle phase: _____ Moon phase: _____

Day/planetary energy: _____ Sun sign: _____

The Feels 🫶

_____

_____

_____

_____

Self-sourcing 🧘

_____

_____

_____

_____

Heart Riffs ✍️

_____

_____

_____

_____

Date: _____ Cycle day: _____

Cycle phase: _____ Moon phase: _____

Day/planetary energy: _____ Sun sign: _____

The Feels 🫶

_____

_____

_____

_____

Self-sourcing 🧘

_____

_____

_____

_____

Heart Riffs ✍️

_____

_____

_____

_____

Date: _____ Cycle day: _____

Cycle phase: _____ Moon phase: _____

Day/planetary energy: _____ Sun sign: _____

The Feels 🫶

_____
_____
_____
_____

Self-sourcing 🧘

_____
_____
_____
_____

Heart Riffs ✍️

_____
_____
_____
_____

Date: _____ Cycle day: _____

Cycle phase: _____ Moon phase: _____

Day/planetary energy: _____ Sun sign: _____

The Feels 🫶

_____
_____
_____
_____

Self-sourcing 🧘

_____
_____
_____
_____

Heart Riffs ✍️

_____
_____
_____
_____

Date: _____ Cycle day: _____

Cycle phase: _____ Moon phase: _____

Day/planetary energy: _____ Sun sign: _____

The Feels 🫱

_____
_____
_____
_____

Self-sourcing 🧘

_____
_____
_____
_____

Heart Riffs ✍️

_____
_____
_____
_____

Date: _____ Cycle day: _____

Cycle phase: _____ Moon phase: _____

Day/planetary energy: _____ Sun sign: _____

The Feels 🫱

_____
_____
_____
_____

Self-sourcing 🧘

_____
_____
_____
_____

Heart Riffs ✍️

_____
_____
_____
_____

Date: Cycle day:

Cycle phase: Moon phase:

Day/planetary energy: Sun sign:

The Feels

_____

_____

_____

_____

Self-sourcing

_____

_____

_____

_____

Heart Riffs

_____

_____

_____

_____

Date: Cycle day:

Cycle phase: Moon phase:

Day/planetary energy: Sun sign:

The Feels

_____

_____

_____

_____

Self-sourcing

_____

_____

_____

_____

Heart Riffs

_____

_____

_____

_____

Date: _____ Cycle day: _____

Cycle phase: _____ Moon phase: _____

Day/planetary energy: _____ Sun sign: _____

The Feels ✋

_____

_____

_____

Self-sourcing 🧘

_____

_____

_____

Heart Riffs ✍

_____

_____

_____

Date: _____ Cycle day: _____

Cycle phase: _____ Moon phase: _____

Day/planetary energy: _____ Sun sign: _____

The Feels ✋

_____

_____

_____

Self-sourcing 🧘

_____

_____

_____

Heart Riffs ✍

_____

_____

_____

Date: _____ Cycle day: _____

Cycle phase: _____ Moon phase: _____

Day/planetary energy: _____ Sun sign: _____

The Feels 🤟

_____

_____

_____

_____

Self-sourcing 🧘

_____

_____

_____

_____

Heart Riffs ✍

_____

_____

_____

_____

Date: _____ Cycle day: _____

Cycle phase: _____ Moon phase: _____

Day/planetary energy: _____ Sun sign: _____

The Feels 🤟

_____

_____

_____

_____

Self-sourcing 🧘

_____

_____

_____

_____

Heart Riffs ✍

_____

_____

_____

_____

Date: _____ Cycle day: _____

Cycle phase: _____ Moon phase: _____

Day/planetary energy: _____ Sun sign: _____

The Feels 🫶

_____

_____

_____

_____

Self-sourcing 🧘

_____

_____

_____

Heart Riffs ✍️

_____

_____

_____

_____

Date: _____ Cycle day: _____

Cycle phase: _____ Moon phase: _____

Day/planetary energy: _____ Sun sign: _____

The Feels 🫶

_____

_____

_____

_____

Self-sourcing 🧘

_____

_____

_____

Heart Riffs ✍️

_____

_____

_____

_____

Date: Cycle day:

Cycle phase: Moon phase:

Day/planetary energy: Sun sign:

The Feels

_____

_____

_____

_____

Self-sourcing

_____

_____

_____

_____

Heart Riffs

_____

_____

_____

_____

Date: Cycle day:

Cycle phase: Moon phase:

Day/planetary energy: Sun sign:

The Feels

_____

_____

_____

_____

Self-sourcing

_____

_____

_____

_____

Heart Riffs

_____

_____

_____

_____

Date: _____ Cycle day: _____
Cycle phase: _____ Moon phase: _____
Day/planetary energy: _____ Sun sign: _____

The Feels 🫶

_____
_____
_____
_____

Self-sourcing 🧘

_____
_____
_____
_____

Heart Riffs ✍️

_____
_____
_____
_____

Date: _____ Cycle day: _____
Cycle phase: _____ Moon phase: _____
Day/planetary energy: _____ Sun sign: _____

The Feels 🫶

_____
_____
_____
_____

Self-sourcing 🧘

_____
_____
_____
_____

Heart Riffs ✍️

_____
_____
_____
_____

Date: Cycle day:

Cycle phase: Moon phase:

Day/planetary energy: Sun sign:

The Feels

_____

_____

_____

Self-sourcing

_____

_____

_____

Heart Riffs

_____

_____

_____

_____

Date: Cycle day:

Cycle phase: Moon phase:

Day/planetary energy: Sun sign:

The Feels

_____

_____

_____

Self-sourcing

_____

_____

_____

Heart Riffs

_____

_____

_____

Date: Cycle day:
Cycle phase: Moon phase:
Day/planetary energy: Sun sign:

The Feels ✋

_____
_____
_____
_____

Self-sourcing 🧘

_____
_____
_____
_____

Heart Riffs ✍

_____
_____
_____
_____

Date: Cycle day:
Cycle phase: Moon phase:
Day/planetary energy: Sun sign:

The Feels ✋

_____
_____
_____
_____

Self-sourcing 🧘

_____
_____
_____
_____

Heart Riffs ✍

_____
_____
_____

Date: _____ Cycle day: _____

Cycle phase: _____ Moon phase: _____

Day/planetary energy: _____ Sun sign: _____

The Feels 🫶

_____

_____

_____

Self-sourcing 🧘

_____

_____

_____

Heart Riffs ✍️

_____

_____

_____

_____

Date: _____ Cycle day: _____

Cycle phase: _____ Moon phase: _____

Day/planetary energy: _____ Sun sign: _____

The Feels 🫶

_____

_____

_____

Self-sourcing 🧘

_____

_____

_____

Heart Riffs ✍️

_____

_____

_____

Date: Cycle day:

Cycle phase: Moon phase:

Day/planetary energy: Sun sign:

The Feels

_____

_____

_____

Self-sourcing

_____

_____

_____

Heart Riffs

_____

_____

_____

_____

Date: Cycle day:

Cycle phase: Moon phase:

Day/planetary energy: Sun sign:

The Feels

_____

_____

_____

Self-sourcing

_____

_____

_____

Heart Riffs

_____

_____

_____

_____

Date: Cycle day:
Cycle phase: Moon phase:
Day/planetary energy: Sun sign:

The Feels 🤲

Self-sourcing 🧘

Heart Riffs ✍️

Date: Cycle day:
Cycle phase: Moon phase:
Day/planetary energy: Sun sign:

The Feels 🤲

Self-sourcing 🧘

Heart Riffs ✍️

Date: _____ Cycle day: _____

Cycle phase: _____ Moon phase: _____

Day/planetary energy: _____ Sun sign: _____

The Feels ✋

_____

_____

_____

_____

Self-sourcing 🧘

_____

_____

_____

Heart Riffs ✍

_____

_____

_____

_____

Date: _____ Cycle day: _____

Cycle phase: _____ Moon phase: _____

Day/planetary energy: _____ Sun sign: _____

The Feels ✋

_____

_____

_____

_____

Self-sourcing 🧘

_____

_____

_____

Heart Riffs ✍

_____

_____

_____

_____

Reflect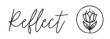

Which cycle days were most positive?

....

....

....

....

....

....

....

Which were most challenging?

....

....

....

....

....

....

....

....

What patterns are unfolding?

....

....

....

....

....

....

....

Notes for your next-cycle self…

....

....

....

....

....

....

....

....

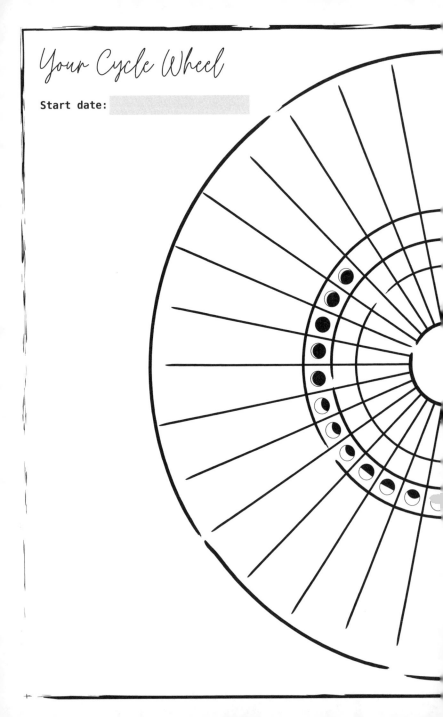

Your Cycle Wheel

Start date:

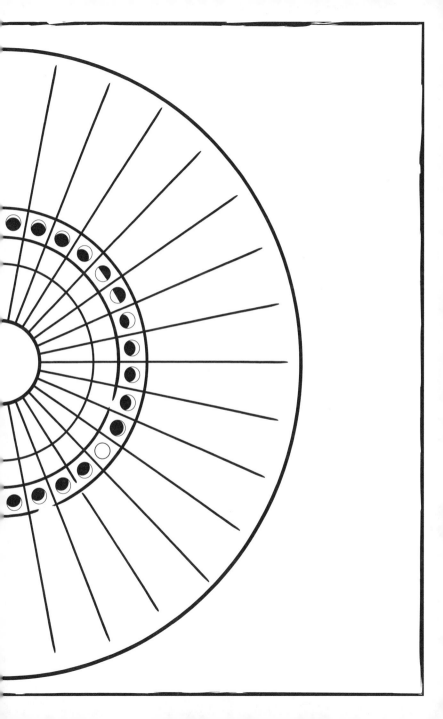

Date: _____   Cycle day: _____
Cycle phase: _____   Moon phase: _____
Day/planetary energy: _____   Sun sign: _____

The Feels 🤲

_____
_____
_____
_____

Self-sourcing 🧘

_____
_____
_____
_____

Heart Riffs ✍️

_____
_____
_____
_____

Date: _____   Cycle day: _____
Cycle phase: _____   Moon phase: _____
Day/planetary energy: _____   Sun sign: _____

The Feels 🤲

_____
_____
_____
_____

Self-sourcing 🧘

_____
_____
_____
_____

Heart Riffs ✍️

_____
_____
_____
_____

Date: ⬚⬚⬚⬚⬚⬚⬚⬚⬚⬚ Cycle day: ⬚⬚⬚⬚⬚⬚

Cycle phase: ⬚⬚⬚⬚⬚⬚⬚⬚ Moon phase: ⬚⬚⬚⬚⬚⬚⬚⬚

Day/planetary energy: ⬚⬚⬚⬚⬚⬚ Sun sign: ⬚⬚⬚⬚⬚

The Feels ✋

_____

_____

_____

_____

Self-sourcing 🧘

_____

_____

_____

_____

Heart Riffs ✍

_____

_____

_____

_____

Date: ⬚⬚⬚⬚⬚⬚⬚⬚⬚⬚ Cycle day: ⬚⬚⬚⬚⬚⬚

Cycle phase: ⬚⬚⬚⬚⬚⬚⬚⬚ Moon phase: ⬚⬚⬚⬚⬚⬚⬚⬚

Day/planetary energy: ⬚⬚⬚⬚⬚⬚ Sun sign: ⬚⬚⬚⬚⬚

The Feels ✋

_____

_____

_____

_____

Self-sourcing 🧘

_____

_____

_____

_____

Heart Riffs ✍

_____

_____

_____

_____

Date: _____ Cycle day: _____

Cycle phase: _____ Moon phase: _____

Day/planetary energy: _____ Sun sign: _____

The Feels 🫶

_____

_____

_____

_____

Self-sourcing 🧘

_____

_____

_____

_____

Heart Riffs ✍️

_____

_____

_____

_____

_____

Date: _____ Cycle day: _____

Cycle phase: _____ Moon phase: _____

Day/planetary energy: _____ Sun sign: _____

The Feels 🫶

_____

_____

_____

_____

Self-sourcing 🧘

_____

_____

_____

_____

Heart Riffs ✍️

_____

_____

_____

_____

Date: _____ Cycle day: _____
Cycle phase: _____ Moon phase: _____
Day/planetary energy: _____ Sun sign: _____

The Feels ✌️

_____
_____
_____
_____

Self-sourcing 🧘

_____
_____
_____
_____

Heart Riffs ✍️

_____
_____
_____
_____

Date: _____ Cycle day: _____
Cycle phase: _____ Moon phase: _____
Day/planetary energy: _____ Sun sign: _____

The Feels ✌️

_____
_____
_____
_____

Self-sourcing 🧘

_____
_____
_____
_____

Heart Riffs ✍️

_____
_____
_____
_____

Date: ⬚⬚⬚⬚⬚ Cycle day: ⬚⬚⬚⬚

Cycle phase: ⬚⬚⬚⬚ Moon phase: ⬚⬚⬚⬚

Day/planetary energy: ⬚⬚⬚⬚ Sun sign: ⬚⬚⬚⬚

The Feels 🫶

_____

_____

_____

_____

Self-sourcing 🧘

_____

_____

_____

_____

Heart Riffs ✍️

_____

_____

_____

_____

Date: ⬚⬚⬚⬚⬚ Cycle day: ⬚⬚⬚⬚

Cycle phase: ⬚⬚⬚⬚ Moon phase: ⬚⬚⬚⬚

Day/planetary energy: ⬚⬚⬚⬚ Sun sign: ⬚⬚⬚⬚

The Feels 🫶

_____

_____

_____

_____

Self-sourcing 🧘

_____

_____

_____

_____

Heart Riffs ✍️

_____

_____

_____

_____

Date: _____ Cycle day: _____

Cycle phase: _____ Moon phase: _____

Day/planetary energy: _____ Sun sign: _____

The Feels 🤲

_____
_____
_____
_____

Self-sourcing 🧘

_____
_____
_____
_____

Heart Riffs ✍️

_____
_____
_____
_____

Date: _____ Cycle day: _____

Cycle phase: _____ Moon phase: _____

Day/planetary energy: _____ Sun sign: _____

The Feels 🤲

_____
_____
_____
_____

Self-sourcing 🧘

_____
_____
_____
_____

Heart Riffs ✍️

_____
_____
_____
_____

Date: _____ Cycle day: _____

Cycle phase: _____ Moon phase: _____

Day/planetary energy: _____ Sun sign: _____

The Feels 🤲

_____

_____

_____

Self-sourcing 🧘

_____

_____

_____

Heart Riffs ✍️

_____

_____

_____

Date: _____ Cycle day: _____

Cycle phase: _____ Moon phase: _____

Day/planetary energy: _____ Sun sign: _____

The Feels 🤲

_____

_____

_____

Self-sourcing 🧘

_____

_____

_____

Heart Riffs ✍️

_____

_____

_____

Date: _____   Cycle day: _____
Cycle phase: _____   Moon phase: _____
Day/planetary energy: _____   Sun sign: _____

The Feels 🫶

_____
_____
_____
_____

Self-sourcing 🧘

_____
_____
_____
_____

Heart Riffs ✍️

_____
_____
_____
_____

Date: _____   Cycle day: _____
Cycle phase: _____   Moon phase: _____
Day/planetary energy: _____   Sun sign: _____

The Feels 🫶

_____
_____
_____
_____

Self-sourcing 🧘

_____
_____
_____
_____

Heart Riffs ✍️

_____
_____
_____
_____

Date: _____   Cycle day: _____

Cycle phase: _____   Moon phase: _____

Day/planetary energy: _____   Sun sign: _____

The Feels ✋

_____

_____

_____

Self-sourcing 🧘

_____

_____

_____

Heart Riffs ✍

_____

_____

_____

_____

Date: _____   Cycle day: _____

Cycle phase: _____   Moon phase: _____

Day/planetary energy: _____   Sun sign: _____

The Feels ✋

_____

_____

_____

Self-sourcing 🧘

_____

_____

_____

Heart Riffs ✍

_____

_____

_____

Date: _____ Cycle day: _____

Cycle phase: _____ Moon phase: _____

Day/planetary energy: _____ Sun sign: _____

The Feels ✋

_____
_____
_____
_____

Self-sourcing 🧘

_____
_____
_____
_____

Heart Riffs ✍

_____
_____
_____
_____

Date: _____ Cycle day: _____

Cycle phase: _____ Moon phase: _____

Day/planetary energy: _____ Sun sign: _____

The Feels ✋

_____
_____
_____
_____

Self-sourcing 🧘

_____
_____
_____
_____

Heart Riffs ✍

_____
_____
_____
_____

Date: _____ Cycle day: _____

Cycle phase: _____ Moon phase: _____

Day/planetary energy: _____ Sun sign: _____

The Feels 🫶

_____

_____

_____

_____

Self-sourcing 🧘

_____

_____

_____

_____

Heart Riffs ✍️

_____

_____

_____

_____

Date: _____ Cycle day: _____

Cycle phase: _____ Moon phase: _____

Day/planetary energy: _____ Sun sign: _____

The Feels 🫶

_____

_____

_____

_____

Self-sourcing 🧘

_____

_____

_____

_____

Heart Riffs ✍️

_____

_____

_____

_____

Date: _____ Cycle day: _____
Cycle phase: _____ Moon phase: _____
Day/planetary energy: _____ Sun sign: _____

The Feels ✋

_____
_____
_____

Self-sourcing 🧘

_____
_____
_____

Heart Riffs ✍

_____
_____
_____
_____

Date: _____ Cycle day: _____
Cycle phase: _____ Moon phase: _____
Day/planetary energy: _____ Sun sign: _____

The Feels ✋

_____
_____
_____

Self-sourcing 🧘

_____
_____
_____

Heart Riffs ✍

_____
_____
_____

Date: _____ Cycle day: _____

Cycle phase: _____ Moon phase: _____

Day/planetary energy: _____ Sun sign: _____

The Feels 🫶

_____

_____

_____

Self-sourcing 🧘

_____

_____

_____

Heart Riffs ✍️

_____

_____

_____

_____

Date: _____ Cycle day: _____

Cycle phase: _____ Moon phase: _____

Day/planetary energy: _____ Sun sign: _____

The Feels 🫶

_____

_____

_____

Self-sourcing 🧘

_____

_____

_____

Heart Riffs ✍️

_____

_____

_____

_____

Date: Cycle day:

Cycle phase: Moon phase:

Day/planetary energy: Sun sign:

The Feels

Self-sourcing

Heart Riffs

Date: Cycle day:

Cycle phase: Moon phase:

Day/planetary energy: Sun sign:

The Feels

Self-sourcing

Heart Riffs

Date: _____   Cycle day: _____

Cycle phase: _____   Moon phase: _____

Day/planetary energy: _____   Sun sign: _____

The Feels 🫶

_____

_____

_____

_____

Self-sourcing 🧘

_____

_____

_____

_____

Heart Riffs ✍️

_____

_____

_____

_____

Date: _____   Cycle day: _____

Cycle phase: _____   Moon phase: _____

Day/planetary energy: _____   Sun sign: _____

The Feels 🫶

_____

_____

_____

_____

Self-sourcing 🧘

_____

_____

_____

_____

Heart Riffs ✍️

_____

_____

_____

_____

Date: _____ Cycle day: _____

Cycle phase: _____ Moon phase: _____

Day/planetary energy: _____ Sun sign: _____

The Feels 🫶

_____

_____

_____

_____

Self-sourcing 🧘

_____

_____

_____

_____

Heart Riffs ✍️

_____

_____

_____

_____

Date: _____ Cycle day: _____

Cycle phase: _____ Moon phase: _____

Day/planetary energy: _____ Sun sign: _____

The Feels 🫶

_____

_____

_____

_____

Self-sourcing 🧘

_____

_____

_____

_____

Heart Riffs ✍️

_____

_____

_____

_____

Reflect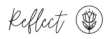

Which cycle days were most positive?

_____

_____

_____

_____

_____

_____

_____

Which were most challenging?

_____

_____

_____

_____

_____

_____

_____

_____

What patterns are unfolding?

....

....

....

....

....

....

....

Notes for your next-cycle self…

....

....

....

....

....

....

....

....

Your Cycle Wheel

Start date:

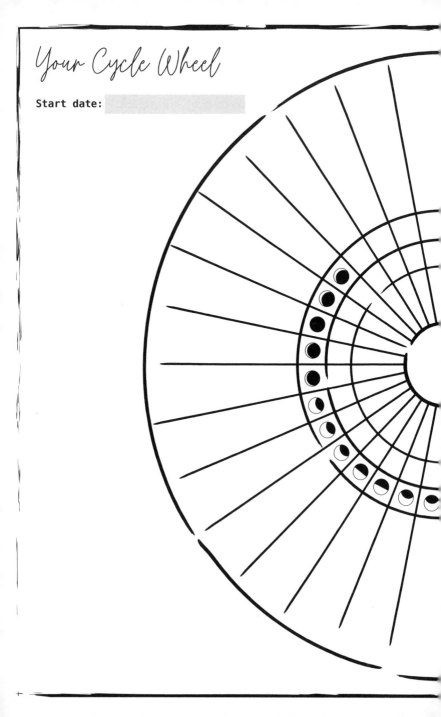

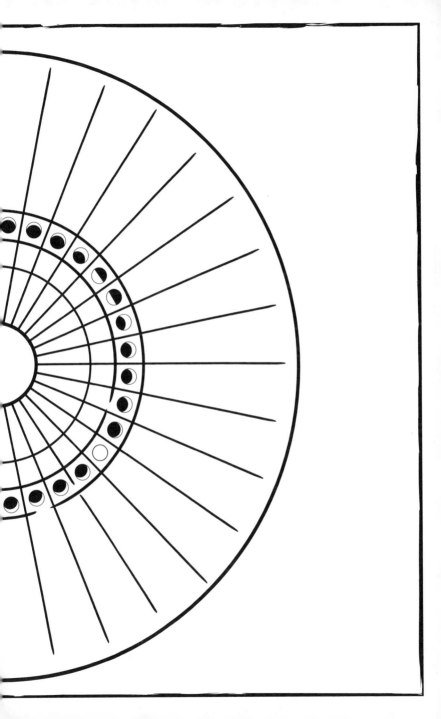

Date: Cycle day:

Cycle phase: Moon phase:

Day/planetary energy: Sun sign:

The Feels

Self-sourcing

Heart Riffs

Date: Cycle day:

Cycle phase: Moon phase:

Day/planetary energy: Sun sign:

The Feels

Self-sourcing

Heart Riffs

Date: Cycle day:

Cycle phase: Moon phase:

Day/planetary energy: Sun sign:

The Feels

Self-sourcing

Heart Riffs

Date: Cycle day:

Cycle phase: Moon phase:

Day/planetary energy: Sun sign:

The Feels

Self-sourcing

Heart Riffs

Date: Cycle day:
Cycle phase: Moon phase:
Day/planetary energy: Sun sign:

The Feels

_____
_____
_____
_____

Self-sourcing

_____
_____
_____
_____

Heart Riffs

_____
_____
_____
_____

Date: Cycle day:
Cycle phase: Moon phase:
Day/planetary energy: Sun sign:

The Feels

_____
_____
_____
_____

Self-sourcing

_____
_____
_____
_____

Heart Riffs

_____
_____
_____
_____

Date: _____ Cycle day: _____

Cycle phase: _____ Moon phase: _____

Day/planetary energy: _____ Sun sign: _____

The Feels 🫶

_____

_____

_____

_____

Self-sourcing 🧘

_____

_____

_____

_____

Heart Riffs ✍️

_____

_____

_____

_____

Date: _____ Cycle day: _____

Cycle phase: _____ Moon phase: _____

Day/planetary energy: _____ Sun sign: _____

The Feels 🫶

_____

_____

_____

_____

Self-sourcing 🧘

_____

_____

_____

_____

Heart Riffs ✍️

_____

_____

_____

_____

Date: Cycle day:

Cycle phase: Moon phase:

Day/planetary energy: Sun sign:

The Feels

_____

_____

_____

Self-sourcing

_____

_____

_____

Heart Riffs

_____

_____

_____

_____

Date: Cycle day:

Cycle phase: Moon phase:

Day/planetary energy: Sun sign:

The Feels

_____

_____

_____

Self-sourcing

_____

_____

_____

Heart Riffs

_____

_____

_____

_____

Date: _____ Cycle day: _____
Cycle phase: _____ Moon phase: _____
Day/planetary energy: _____ Sun sign: _____

The Feels 🤲

_____
_____
_____
_____

Self-sourcing 🧘

_____
_____
_____
_____

Heart Riffs ✍️

_____
_____
_____
_____

Date: _____ Cycle day: _____
Cycle phase: _____ Moon phase: _____
Day/planetary energy: _____ Sun sign: _____

The Feels 🤲

_____
_____
_____
_____

Self-sourcing 🧘

_____
_____
_____
_____

Heart Riffs ✍️

_____
_____
_____
_____

Date: Cycle day:

Cycle phase: Moon phase:

Day/planetary energy: Sun sign:

The Feels

Self-sourcing

Heart Riffs

Date: Cycle day:

Cycle phase: Moon phase:

Day/planetary energy: Sun sign:

The Feels

Self-sourcing

Heart Riffs

Date: Cycle day:

Cycle phase: Moon phase:

Day/planetary energy: Sun sign:

The Feels

Self-sourcing

Heart Riffs

Date: Cycle day:

Cycle phase: Moon phase:

Day/planetary energy: Sun sign:

The Feels

Self-sourcing

Heart Riffs

Date: Cycle day:

Cycle phase: Moon phase:

Day/planetary energy: Sun sign:

The Feels 🫶

_____

_____

_____

Self-sourcing 🧘

_____

_____

_____

Heart Riffs ✍️

_____

_____

_____

_____

Date: Cycle day:

Cycle phase: Moon phase:

Day/planetary energy: Sun sign:

The Feels 🫶

_____

_____

_____

Self-sourcing 🧘

_____

_____

_____

Heart Riffs ✍️

_____

_____

_____

Date: _____ Cycle day: _____
Cycle phase: _____ Moon phase: _____
Day/planetary energy: _____ Sun sign: _____

The Feels 🫶

_____
_____
_____
_____

Self-sourcing 🧘

_____
_____
_____
_____

Heart Riffs ✍️

_____
_____
_____
_____

Date: _____ Cycle day: _____
Cycle phase: _____ Moon phase: _____
Day/planetary energy: _____ Sun sign: _____

The Feels 🫶

_____
_____
_____
_____

Self-sourcing 🧘

_____
_____
_____
_____

Heart Riffs ✍️

_____
_____
_____
_____

Date: _____ Cycle day: _____

Cycle phase: _____ Moon phase: _____

Day/planetary energy: _____ Sun sign: _____

The Feels 🖐️

_____

_____

_____

_____

Self-sourcing 🧘

_____

_____

_____

Heart Riffs ✍️

_____

_____

_____

_____

Date: _____ Cycle day: _____

Cycle phase: _____ Moon phase: _____

Day/planetary energy: _____ Sun sign: _____

The Feels 🖐️

_____

_____

_____

_____

Self-sourcing 🧘

_____

_____

_____

Heart Riffs ✍️

_____

_____

_____

_____

Date: _____ Cycle day: _____

Cycle phase: _____ Moon phase: _____

Day/planetary energy: _____ Sun sign: _____

The Feels ✋

_____

_____

_____

_____

Self-sourcing 🧘

_____

_____

_____

Heart Riffs ✍

_____

_____

_____

_____

Date: _____ Cycle day: _____

Cycle phase: _____ Moon phase: _____

Day/planetary energy: _____ Sun sign: _____

The Feels ✋

_____

_____

_____

_____

Self-sourcing 🧘

_____

_____

_____

Heart Riffs ✍

_____

_____

_____

_____

Date: [_____] Cycle day: [_____]
Cycle phase: [_____] Moon phase: [_____]
Day/planetary energy: [_____] Sun sign: [_____]

The Feels 🫶

_____
_____
_____
_____

Self-sourcing 🧘

_____
_____
_____
_____

Heart Riffs ✍️

_____
_____
_____
_____

Date: [_____] Cycle day: [_____]
Cycle phase: [_____] Moon phase: [_____]
Day/planetary energy: [_____] Sun sign: [_____]

The Feels 🫶

_____
_____
_____
_____

Self-sourcing 🧘

_____
_____
_____
_____

Heart Riffs ✍️

_____
_____
_____
_____

Date: _____ Cycle day: _____

Cycle phase: _____ Moon phase: _____

Day/planetary energy: _____ Sun sign: _____

The Feels 🫶

_____

_____

_____

Self-sourcing 🧘

_____

_____

_____

Heart Riffs ✍️

_____

_____

_____

Date: _____ Cycle day: _____

Cycle phase: _____ Moon phase: _____

Day/planetary energy: _____ Sun sign: _____

The Feels 🫶

_____

_____

_____

Self-sourcing 🧘

_____

_____

_____

Heart Riffs ✍️

_____

_____

_____

Date: _____ Cycle day: _____
Cycle phase: _____ Moon phase: _____
Day/planetary energy: _____ Sun sign: _____

The Feels 🫶

_____
_____
_____
_____

Self-sourcing 🧘

_____
_____
_____
_____

Heart Riffs ✍️

_____
_____
_____
_____

Date: _____ Cycle day: _____
Cycle phase: _____ Moon phase: _____
Day/planetary energy: _____ Sun sign: _____

The Feels 🫶

_____
_____
_____
_____

Self-sourcing 🧘

_____
_____
_____
_____

Heart Riffs ✍️

_____
_____
_____
_____

Date: _____ Cycle day: _____

Cycle phase: _____ Moon phase: _____

Day/planetary energy: _____ Sun sign: _____

The Feels ✋

_____

_____

_____

_____

Self-sourcing 🧘

_____

_____

_____

_____

Heart Riffs ✍

_____

_____

_____

_____

Date: _____ Cycle day: _____

Cycle phase: _____ Moon phase: _____

Day/planetary energy: _____ Sun sign: _____

The Feels ✋

_____

_____

_____

_____

Self-sourcing 🧘

_____

_____

_____

_____

Heart Riffs ✍

_____

_____

_____

_____

Reflect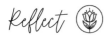

Which cycle days were most positive?

_____

_____

_____

_____

_____

_____

_____

_____

Which were most challenging?

_____

_____

_____

_____

_____

_____

_____

_____

_____

What patterns are unfolding?

Notes for your next-cycle self...

Your Cycle Wheel

Start date:

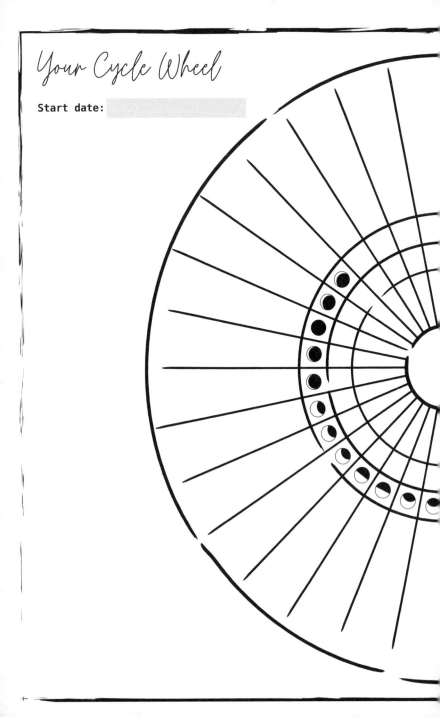

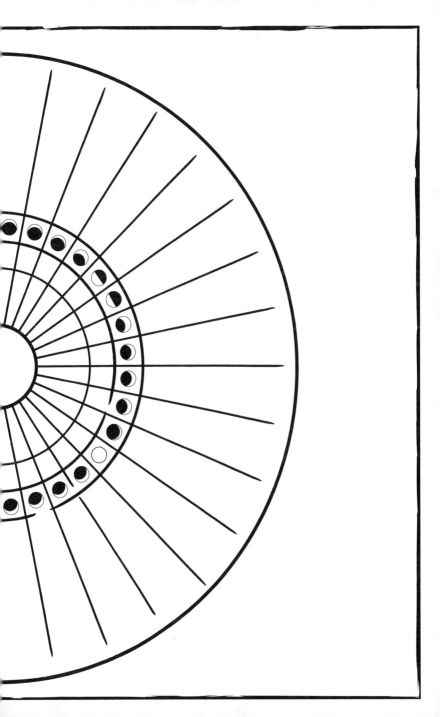

Date: _____ Cycle day: _____

Cycle phase: _____ Moon phase: _____

Day/planetary energy: _____ Sun sign: _____

The Feels ✋

_____

_____

_____

Self-sourcing 🧘

_____

_____

_____

Heart Riffs ✍

_____

_____

_____

_____

Date: _____ Cycle day: _____

Cycle phase: _____ Moon phase: _____

Day/planetary energy: _____ Sun sign: _____

The Feels ✋

_____

_____

_____

Self-sourcing 🧘

_____

_____

_____

Heart Riffs ✍

_____

_____

_____

Date: _____ Cycle day: _____
Cycle phase: _____ Moon phase: _____
Day/planetary energy: _____ Sun sign: _____

The Feels 🫶

_____
_____
_____
_____

Self-sourcing 🧘

_____
_____
_____
_____

Heart Riffs ✍️

_____
_____
_____
_____

Date: _____ Cycle day: _____
Cycle phase: _____ Moon phase: _____
Day/planetary energy: _____ Sun sign: _____

The Feels 🫶

_____
_____
_____
_____

Self-sourcing 🧘

_____
_____
_____
_____

Heart Riffs ✍️

_____
_____
_____
_____

Date: _____ Cycle day: _____
Cycle phase: _____ Moon phase: _____
Day/planetary energy: _____ Sun sign: _____

The Feels ✋

_____
_____
_____

Self-sourcing 🧘

_____
_____
_____
_____

Heart Riffs ✍

_____
_____
_____
_____

Date: _____ Cycle day: _____
Cycle phase: _____ Moon phase: _____
Day/planetary energy: _____ Sun sign: _____

The Feels ✋

_____
_____
_____

Self-sourcing 🧘

_____
_____
_____
_____

Heart Riffs ✍

_____
_____
_____

Date: _____ Cycle day: _____

Cycle phase: _____ Moon phase: _____

Day/planetary energy: _____ Sun sign: _____

The Feels

_____

_____

_____

Self-sourcing

_____

_____

_____

Heart Riffs

_____

_____

_____

_____

Date: _____ Cycle day: _____

Cycle phase: _____ Moon phase: _____

Day/planetary energy: _____ Sun sign: _____

The Feels

_____

_____

_____

Self-sourcing

_____

_____

_____

Heart Riffs

_____

_____

_____

_____

Date: Cycle day:

Cycle phase: Moon phase:

Day/planetary energy: Sun sign:

The Feels 🤲

Self-sourcing 🧘

Heart Riffs ✍️

Date: Cycle day:

Cycle phase: Moon phase:

Day/planetary energy: Sun sign:

The Feels 🤲

Self-sourcing 🧘

Heart Riffs ✍️

Date: ⬚ Cycle day: ⬚
Cycle phase: ⬚ Moon phase: ⬚
Day/planetary energy: ⬚ Sun sign: ⬚

The Feels 🫰

_____
_____
_____
_____

Self-sourcing 🧘

_____
_____
_____
_____

Heart Riffs ✍

_____
_____
_____
_____

Date: ⬚ Cycle day: ⬚
Cycle phase: ⬚ Moon phase: ⬚
Day/planetary energy: ⬚ Sun sign: ⬚

The Feels 🫰

_____
_____
_____
_____

Self-sourcing 🧘

_____
_____
_____
_____

Heart Riffs ✍

_____
_____
_____
_____

Date: _____ Cycle day: _____

Cycle phase: _____ Moon phase: _____

Day/planetary energy: _____ Sun sign: _____

The Feels 🤲

_____
_____
_____
_____

Self-sourcing 🧘

_____
_____
_____
_____

Heart Riffs ✍️

_____
_____
_____
_____

Date: _____ Cycle day: _____

Cycle phase: _____ Moon phase: _____

Day/planetary energy: _____ Sun sign: _____

The Feels 🤲

_____
_____
_____
_____

Self-sourcing 🧘

_____
_____
_____
_____

Heart Riffs ✍️

_____
_____
_____
_____

Date: Cycle day:

Cycle phase: Moon phase:

Day/planetary energy: Sun sign:

The Feels

_____

_____

_____

_____

Self-sourcing

_____

_____

_____

_____

Heart Riffs

_____

_____

_____

_____

Date: Cycle day:

Cycle phase: Moon phase:

Day/planetary energy: Sun sign:

The Feels

_____

_____

_____

_____

Self-sourcing

_____

_____

_____

_____

Heart Riffs

_____

_____

_____

_____

Date: Cycle day:

Cycle phase: Moon phase:

Day/planetary energy: Sun sign:

The Feels

_____

_____

_____

Self-sourcing

_____

_____

_____

Heart Riffs

_____

_____

_____

_____

Date: Cycle day:

Cycle phase: Moon phase:

Day/planetary energy: Sun sign:

The Feels

_____

_____

_____

Self-sourcing

_____

_____

_____

Heart Riffs

_____

_____

_____

Date: _____ Cycle day: _____

Cycle phase: _____ Moon phase: _____

Day/planetary energy: _____ Sun sign: _____

The Feels 🫶

_____
_____
_____
_____

Self-sourcing 🧘

_____
_____
_____
_____

Heart Riffs ✍

_____
_____
_____
_____

Date: _____ Cycle day: _____

Cycle phase: _____ Moon phase: _____

Day/planetary energy: _____ Sun sign: _____

The Feels 🫶

_____
_____
_____
_____

Self-sourcing 🧘

_____
_____
_____
_____

Heart Riffs ✍

_____
_____
_____
_____

Date: _____ Cycle day: _____

Cycle phase: _____ Moon phase: _____

Day/planetary energy: _____ Sun sign: _____

The Feels 🫰

_____

_____

_____

_____

Self-sourcing 🧘

_____

_____

_____

_____

Heart Riffs ✍️

_____

_____

_____

_____

Date: _____ Cycle day: _____

Cycle phase: _____ Moon phase: _____

Day/planetary energy: _____ Sun sign: _____

The Feels 🫰

_____

_____

_____

_____

Self-sourcing 🧘

_____

_____

_____

_____

Heart Riffs ✍️

_____

_____

_____

_____

Date: Cycle day:
Cycle phase: Moon phase:
Day/planetary energy: Sun sign:

The Feels 🫶

_____
_____
_____

Self-sourcing 🧘

_____
_____
_____

Heart Riffs ✍️

_____
_____
_____

Date: Cycle day:
Cycle phase: Moon phase:
Day/planetary energy: Sun sign:

The Feels 🫶

_____
_____
_____

Self-sourcing 🧘

_____
_____
_____

Heart Riffs ✍️

_____
_____
_____

Date: Cycle day:

Cycle phase: Moon phase:

Day/planetary energy: Sun sign:

The Feels

_____

_____

_____

Self-sourcing

_____

_____

_____

Heart Riffs

_____

_____

_____

_____

Date: Cycle day:

Cycle phase: Moon phase:

Day/planetary energy: Sun sign:

The Feels

_____

_____

_____

Self-sourcing

_____

_____

_____

Heart Riffs

_____

_____

_____

Date: Cycle day:

Cycle phase: Moon phase:

Day/planetary energy: Sun sign:

The Feels

_____

_____

_____

Self-sourcing

_____

_____

_____

Heart Riffs

_____

_____

_____

_____

Date: Cycle day:

Cycle phase: Moon phase:

Day/planetary energy: Sun sign:

The Feels

_____

_____

_____

Self-sourcing

_____

_____

_____

Heart Riffs

_____

_____

_____

Date: Cycle day:

Cycle phase: Moon phase:

Day/planetary energy: Sun sign:

The Feels 🫶

Self-sourcing 🧘

Heart Riffs ✍

Date: Cycle day:

Cycle phase: Moon phase:

Day/planetary energy: Sun sign:

The Feels 🫶

Self-sourcing 🧘

Heart Riffs ✍

Date: _____ Cycle day: _____

Cycle phase: _____ Moon phase: _____

Day/planetary energy: _____ Sun sign: _____

The Feels 🫶

_____

_____

_____

_____

Self-sourcing 🧘

_____

_____

_____

Heart Riffs ✍️

_____

_____

_____

_____

Date: _____ Cycle day: _____

Cycle phase: _____ Moon phase: _____

Day/planetary energy: _____ Sun sign: _____

The Feels 🫶

_____

_____

_____

_____

Self-sourcing 🧘

_____

_____

_____

Heart Riffs ✍️

_____

_____

_____

_____

Reflect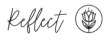

Which cycle days were most positive?

_____

_____

_____

_____

_____

_____

Which were most challenging?

_____

_____

_____

_____

_____

_____

_____

_____

What patterns are unfolding?

....

....

....

....

....

....

Notes for your next-cycle self...

....

....

....

....

....

....

....

....

Your Cycle Wheel

Start date:

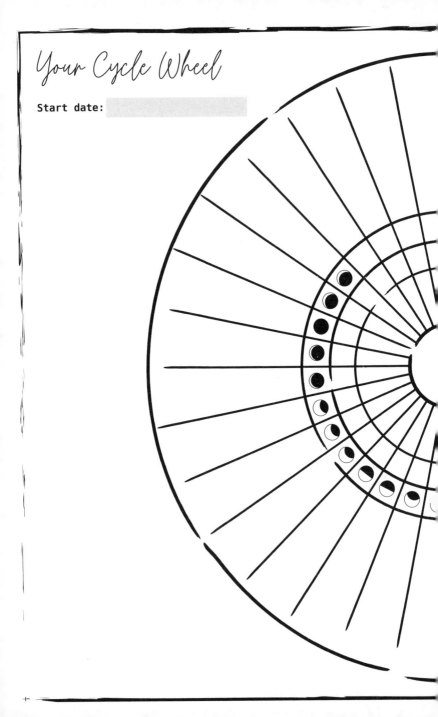

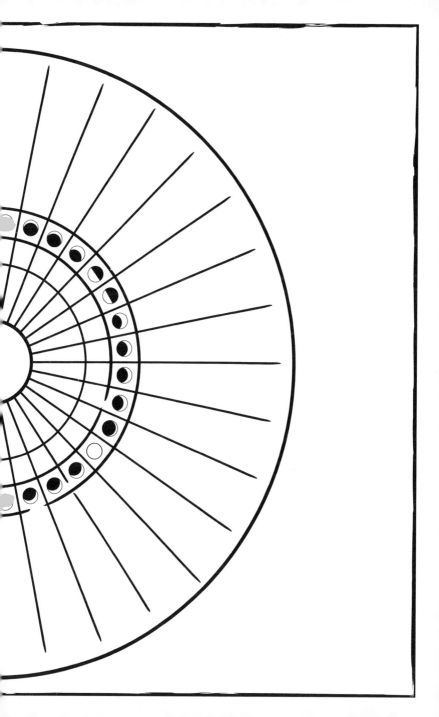

Date: Cycle day:

Cycle phase: Moon phase:

Day/planetary energy: Sun sign:

The Feels 🫶

_____

_____

_____

_____

Self-sourcing 🧘

_____

_____

_____

Heart Riffs ✍️

_____

_____

_____

_____

Date: Cycle day:

Cycle phase: Moon phase:

Day/planetary energy: Sun sign:

The Feels 🫶

_____

_____

_____

_____

Self-sourcing 🧘

_____

_____

_____

Heart Riffs ✍️

_____

_____

_____

_____

Date: _____ Cycle day: _____
Cycle phase: _____ Moon phase: _____
Day/planetary energy: _____ Sun sign: _____

The Feels ✋

_____
_____
_____
_____

Self-sourcing 🧘

_____
_____
_____
_____

Heart Riffs ✍

_____
_____
_____
_____

Date: _____ Cycle day: _____
Cycle phase: _____ Moon phase: _____
Day/planetary energy: _____ Sun sign: _____

The Feels ✋

_____
_____
_____
_____

Self-sourcing 🧘

_____
_____
_____
_____

Heart Riffs ✍

_____
_____
_____
_____

Date: _____   Cycle day: _____

Cycle phase: _____   Moon phase: _____

Day/planetary energy: _____   Sun sign: _____

The Feels 🫶

_____

_____

_____

_____

Self-sourcing 🧘

_____

_____

_____

_____

Heart Riffs ✍️

_____

_____

_____

_____

Date: _____   Cycle day: _____

Cycle phase: _____   Moon phase: _____

Day/planetary energy: _____   Sun sign: _____

The Feels 🫶

_____

_____

_____

_____

Self-sourcing 🧘

_____

_____

_____

_____

Heart Riffs ✍️

_____

_____

_____

_____

Date: Cycle day:

Cycle phase: Moon phase:

Day/planetary energy: Sun sign:

The Feels 🫶

_____

_____

_____

Self-sourcing 🧘

_____

_____

_____

Heart Riffs ✍

_____

_____

_____

_____

Date: Cycle day:

Cycle phase: Moon phase:

Day/planetary energy: Sun sign:

The Feels 🫶

_____

_____

_____

Self-sourcing 🧘

_____

_____

_____

Heart Riffs ✍

_____

_____

_____

_____

Date: Cycle day:

Cycle phase: Moon phase:

Day/planetary energy: Sun sign:

The Feels

_____

_____

_____

_____

Self-sourcing

_____

_____

_____

_____

Heart Riffs

_____

_____

_____

_____

Date: Cycle day:

Cycle phase: Moon phase:

Day/planetary energy: Sun sign:

The Feels

_____

_____

_____

_____

Self-sourcing

_____

_____

_____

_____

Heart Riffs

_____

_____

_____

_____

Date: _____ Cycle day: _____

Cycle phase: _____ Moon phase: _____

Day/planetary energy: _____ Sun sign: _____

The Feels 🤲

_____
_____
_____
_____

Self-sourcing 🧘

_____
_____
_____
_____

Heart Riffs ✍️

_____
_____
_____
_____

Date: _____ Cycle day: _____

Cycle phase: _____ Moon phase: _____

Day/planetary energy: _____ Sun sign: _____

The Feels 🤲

_____
_____
_____
_____

Self-sourcing 🧘

_____
_____
_____
_____

Heart Riffs ✍️

_____
_____
_____
_____

Date: Cycle day:

Cycle phase: Moon phase:

Day/planetary energy: Sun sign:

The Feels 🫶

_____

_____

_____

Self-sourcing 🧘

_____

_____

_____

Heart Riffs ✍️

_____

_____

_____

Date: Cycle day:

Cycle phase: Moon phase:

Day/planetary energy: Sun sign:

The Feels 🫶

_____

_____

_____

Self-sourcing 🧘

_____

_____

_____

Heart Riffs ✍️

_____

_____

_____

Date: _____ Cycle day: _____

Cycle phase: _____ Moon phase: _____

Day/planetary energy: _____ Sun sign: _____

The Feels ⊕

_____

_____

_____

_____

Self-sourcing ⊛

_____

_____

_____

_____

Heart Riffs ✎

_____

_____

_____

_____

Date: _____ Cycle day: _____

Cycle phase: _____ Moon phase: _____

Day/planetary energy: _____ Sun sign: _____

The Feels ⊕

_____

_____

_____

_____

Self-sourcing ⊛

_____

_____

_____

_____

Heart Riffs ✎

_____

_____

_____

_____

Date: _____ Cycle day: _____

Cycle phase: _____ Moon phase: _____

Day/planetary energy: _____ Sun sign: _____

The Feels 🫶

_____

_____

_____

Self-sourcing 🧘

_____

_____

_____

Heart Riffs ✍️

_____

_____

_____

_____

Date: _____ Cycle day: _____

Cycle phase: _____ Moon phase: _____

Day/planetary energy: _____ Sun sign: _____

The Feels 🫶

_____

_____

_____

Self-sourcing 🧘

_____

_____

_____

Heart Riffs ✍️

_____

_____

_____

_____

Date: _____ Cycle day: _____

Cycle phase: _____ Moon phase: _____

Day/planetary energy: _____ Sun sign: _____

The Feels ✋

_____

_____

_____

Self-sourcing 🧘

_____

_____

_____

Heart Riffs ✍

_____

_____

_____

Date: _____ Cycle day: _____

Cycle phase: _____ Moon phase: _____

Day/planetary energy: _____ Sun sign: _____

The Feels ✋

_____

_____

_____

Self-sourcing 🧘

_____

_____

_____

Heart Riffs ✍

_____

_____

_____

Date: _____ Cycle day: _____

Cycle phase: _____ Moon phase: _____

Day/planetary energy: _____ Sun sign: _____

The Feels 🫶

_____

_____

_____

_____

Self-sourcing 🧘

_____

_____

_____

Heart Riffs ✍️

_____

_____

_____

_____

Date: _____ Cycle day: _____

Cycle phase: _____ Moon phase: _____

Day/planetary energy: _____ Sun sign: _____

The Feels 🫶

_____

_____

_____

_____

Self-sourcing 🧘

_____

_____

_____

Heart Riffs ✍️

_____

_____

_____

_____

Date: Cycle day:

Cycle phase: Moon phase:

Day/planetary energy: Sun sign:

The Feels

_____

_____

_____

_____

Self-sourcing

_____

_____

_____

_____

Heart Riffs

_____

_____

_____

_____

Date: Cycle day:

Cycle phase: Moon phase:

Day/planetary energy: Sun sign:

The Feels

_____

_____

_____

_____

Self-sourcing

_____

_____

_____

_____

Heart Riffs

_____

_____

_____

_____

Date: _____ Cycle day: _____

Cycle phase: _____ Moon phase: _____

Day/planetary energy: _____ Sun sign: _____

The Feels 🫶

_____

_____

_____

Self-sourcing 🧘

_____

_____

_____

Heart Riffs ✍️

_____

_____

_____

Date: _____ Cycle day: _____

Cycle phase: _____ Moon phase: _____

Day/planetary energy: _____ Sun sign: _____

The Feels 🫶

_____

_____

_____

Self-sourcing 🧘

_____

_____

_____

Heart Riffs ✍️

_____

_____

_____

Date: _____ Cycle day: _____

Cycle phase: _____ Moon phase: _____

Day/planetary energy: _____ Sun sign: _____

The Feels 🫶

_____

_____

_____

Self-sourcing 🧘

_____

_____

_____

Heart Riffs ✍️

_____

_____

_____

_____

Date: _____ Cycle day: _____

Cycle phase: _____ Moon phase: _____

Day/planetary energy: _____ Sun sign: _____

The Feels 🫶

_____

_____

_____

Self-sourcing 🧘

_____

_____

_____

Heart Riffs ✍️

_____

_____

_____

_____

Date: _____ Cycle day: _____

Cycle phase: _____ Moon phase: _____

Day/planetary energy: _____ Sun sign: _____

The Feels 🤲

_____

_____

_____

Self-sourcing 🧘

_____

_____

_____

Heart Riffs ✍️

_____

_____

_____

_____

Date: _____ Cycle day: _____

Cycle phase: _____ Moon phase: _____

Day/planetary energy: _____ Sun sign: _____

The Feels 🤲

_____

_____

_____

Self-sourcing 🧘

_____

_____

_____

Heart Riffs ✍️

_____

_____

_____

_____

Date: Cycle day:

Cycle phase: Moon phase:

Day/planetary energy: Sun sign:

The Feels

Self-sourcing

Heart Riffs

Date: Cycle day:

Cycle phase: Moon phase:

Day/planetary energy: Sun sign:

The Feels

Self-sourcing

Heart Riffs

Reflect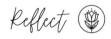

Which cycle days were most positive?

....

....

....

....

....

....

....

Which were most challenging?

....

....

....

....

....

....

....

....

What patterns are unfolding?

Notes for your next-cycle self...

Your Cycle Wheel

Start date:

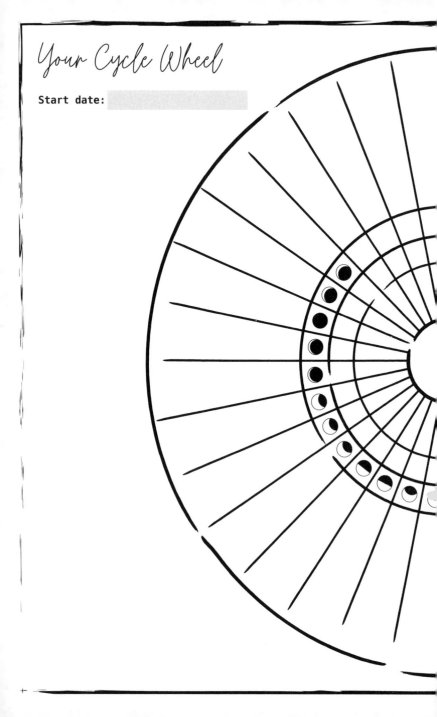

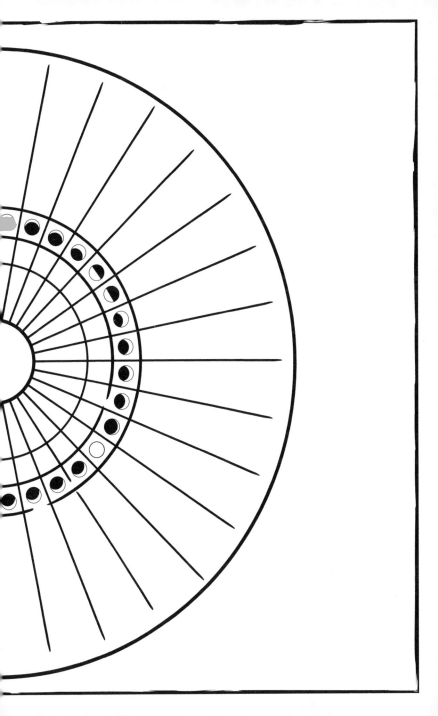

Date: _____ Cycle day: _____

Cycle phase: _____ Moon phase: _____

Day/planetary energy: _____ Sun sign: _____

The Feels 🫶

_____
_____
_____
_____

Self-sourcing 🧘

_____
_____
_____
_____

Heart Riffs ✍️

_____
_____
_____
_____

Date: _____ Cycle day: _____

Cycle phase: _____ Moon phase: _____

Day/planetary energy: _____ Sun sign: _____

The Feels 🫶

_____
_____
_____
_____

Self-sourcing 🧘

_____
_____
_____
_____

Heart Riffs ✍️

_____
_____
_____
_____

Date: Cycle day:

Cycle phase: Moon phase:

Day/planetary energy: Sun sign:

The Feels

_____

_____

_____

_____

Self-sourcing

_____

_____

_____

_____

Heart Riffs

_____

_____

_____

_____

Date: Cycle day:

Cycle phase: Moon phase:

Day/planetary energy: Sun sign:

The Feels

_____

_____

_____

_____

Self-sourcing

_____

_____

_____

_____

Heart Riffs

_____

_____

_____

_____

Date: ⬚⬚⬚⬚⬚⬚⬚⬚⬚⬚⬚⬚ Cycle day: ⬚⬚⬚⬚⬚⬚

Cycle phase: ⬚⬚⬚⬚⬚⬚⬚⬚⬚ Moon phase: ⬚⬚⬚⬚⬚⬚⬚⬚⬚⬚

Day/planetary energy: ⬚⬚⬚⬚⬚⬚⬚⬚ Sun sign: ⬚⬚⬚⬚⬚⬚

The Feels 🫶

_____

_____

_____

_____

Self-sourcing 🧘

_____

_____

_____

_____

Heart Riffs ✍️

_____

_____

_____

_____

Date: ⬚⬚⬚⬚⬚⬚⬚⬚⬚⬚⬚⬚ Cycle day: ⬚⬚⬚⬚⬚⬚

Cycle phase: ⬚⬚⬚⬚⬚⬚⬚⬚⬚ Moon phase: ⬚⬚⬚⬚⬚⬚⬚⬚⬚⬚

Day/planetary energy: ⬚⬚⬚⬚⬚⬚⬚⬚ Sun sign: ⬚⬚⬚⬚⬚⬚

The Feels 🫶

_____

_____

_____

_____

Self-sourcing 🧘

_____

_____

_____

_____

Heart Riffs ✍️

_____

_____

_____

_____

Date: _____   Cycle day: _____
Cycle phase: _____   Moon phase: _____
Day/planetary energy: _____   Sun sign: _____

The Feels ☺

_____
_____
_____
_____

Self-sourcing ☺

_____
_____
_____
_____

Heart Riffs ✍

_____
_____
_____
_____

Date: _____   Cycle day: _____
Cycle phase: _____   Moon phase: _____
Day/planetary energy: _____   Sun sign: _____

The Feels ☺

_____
_____
_____
_____

Self-sourcing ☺

_____
_____
_____
_____

Heart Riffs ✍

_____
_____
_____

Date: Cycle day:
Cycle phase: Moon phase:
Day/planetary energy: Sun sign:

The Feels

_____
_____
_____
_____

Self-sourcing

_____
_____
_____
_____

Heart Riffs

_____
_____
_____
_____

Date: Cycle day:
Cycle phase: Moon phase:
Day/planetary energy: Sun sign:

The Feels

_____
_____
_____
_____

Self-sourcing

_____
_____
_____
_____

Heart Riffs

_____
_____
_____

Date: Cycle day:

Cycle phase: Moon phase:

Day/planetary energy: Sun sign:

The Feels

Self-sourcing

Heart Riffs

Date: Cycle day:

Cycle phase: Moon phase:

Day/planetary energy: Sun sign:

The Feels

Self-sourcing

Heart Riffs

Date: _____ Cycle day: _____

Cycle phase: _____ Moon phase: _____

Day/planetary energy: _____ Sun sign: _____

The Feels 🫶

_____

_____

_____

_____

Self-sourcing 🧘

_____

_____

_____

_____

Heart Riffs ✍️

_____

_____

_____

_____

Date: _____ Cycle day: _____

Cycle phase: _____ Moon phase: _____

Day/planetary energy: _____ Sun sign: _____

The Feels 🫶

_____

_____

_____

_____

Self-sourcing 🧘

_____

_____

_____

_____

Heart Riffs ✍️

_____

_____

_____

_____

Date: Cycle day:

Cycle phase: Moon phase:

Day/planetary energy: Sun sign:

The Feels

Self-sourcing

Heart Riffs

Date: Cycle day:

Cycle phase: Moon phase:

Day/planetary energy: Sun sign:

The Feels

Self-sourcing

Heart Riffs

Date: _____ Cycle day: _____

Cycle phase: _____ Moon phase: _____

Day/planetary energy: _____ Sun sign: _____

The Feels

_____
_____
_____
_____

Self-sourcing

_____
_____
_____
_____

Heart Riffs

_____
_____
_____
_____

Date: _____ Cycle day: _____

Cycle phase: _____ Moon phase: _____

Day/planetary energy: _____ Sun sign: _____

The Feels

_____
_____
_____
_____

Self-sourcing

_____
_____
_____
_____

Heart Riffs

_____
_____
_____
_____

Date: _____   Cycle day: _____
Cycle phase: _____   Moon phase: _____
Day/planetary energy: _____   Sun sign: _____

The Feels

_____
_____
_____
_____

Self-sourcing

_____
_____
_____
_____

Heart Riffs

_____
_____
_____
_____

Date: _____   Cycle day: _____
Cycle phase: _____   Moon phase: _____
Day/planetary energy: _____   Sun sign: _____

The Feels

_____
_____
_____
_____

Self-sourcing

_____
_____
_____
_____

Heart Riffs

_____
_____
_____
_____

Date: Cycle day:

Cycle phase: Moon phase:

Day/planetary energy: Sun sign:

The Feels

Self-sourcing

Heart Riffs

Date: Cycle day:

Cycle phase: Moon phase:

Day/planetary energy: Sun sign:

The Feels

Self-sourcing

Heart Riffs

Date: _____ Cycle day: _____
Cycle phase: _____ Moon phase: _____
Day/planetary energy: _____ Sun sign: _____

The Feels 🫶

_____
_____
_____
_____

Self-sourcing 🧘

_____
_____
_____
_____

Heart Riffs ✍️

_____
_____
_____
_____

Date: _____ Cycle day: _____
Cycle phase: _____ Moon phase: _____
Day/planetary energy: _____ Sun sign: _____

The Feels 🫶

_____
_____
_____
_____

Self-sourcing 🧘

_____
_____
_____
_____

Heart Riffs ✍️

_____
_____
_____
_____

Date: Cycle day:

Cycle phase: Moon phase:

Day/planetary energy: Sun sign:

The Feels

_____

_____

_____

_____

Self-sourcing

_____

_____

_____

Heart Riffs

_____

_____

_____

_____

Date: Cycle day:

Cycle phase: Moon phase:

Day/planetary energy: Sun sign:

The Feels

_____

_____

_____

_____

Self-sourcing

_____

_____

_____

Heart Riffs

_____

_____

_____

_____

Date: _____ Cycle day: _____
Cycle phase: _____ Moon phase: _____
Day/planetary energy: _____ Sun sign: _____

The Feels

_____
_____
_____
_____

Self-sourcing

_____
_____
_____
_____

Heart Riffs

_____
_____
_____
_____

Date: _____ Cycle day: _____
Cycle phase: _____ Moon phase: _____
Day/planetary energy: _____ Sun sign: _____

The Feels

_____
_____
_____
_____

Self-sourcing

_____
_____
_____
_____

Heart Riffs

_____
_____
_____
_____

Date: _____ Cycle day: _____
Cycle phase: _____ Moon phase: _____
Day/planetary energy: _____ Sun sign: _____

The Feels 🫶

_____
_____
_____
_____

Self-sourcing 🧘

_____
_____
_____
_____

Heart Riffs ✍️

_____
_____
_____
_____

Date: _____ Cycle day: _____
Cycle phase: _____ Moon phase: _____
Day/planetary energy: _____ Sun sign: _____

The Feels 🫶

_____
_____
_____
_____

Self-sourcing 🧘

_____
_____
_____
_____

Heart Riffs ✍️

_____
_____
_____
_____

Date: _____ Cycle day: _____
Cycle phase: _____ Moon phase: _____
Day/planetary energy: _____ Sun sign: _____

The Feels

_____
_____
_____
_____

Self-sourcing

_____
_____
_____
_____

Heart Riffs

_____
_____
_____
_____

Date: _____ Cycle day: _____
Cycle phase: _____ Moon phase: _____
Day/planetary energy: _____ Sun sign: _____

The Feels

_____
_____
_____
_____

Self-sourcing

_____
_____
_____
_____

Heart Riffs

_____
_____
_____
_____

Reflect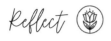

Which cycle days were most positive?

_____

_____

_____

_____

_____

_____

_____

Which were most challenging?

_____

_____

_____

_____

_____

_____

_____

_____

What patterns are unfolding?

....

....

....

....

....

....

....

Notes for your next-cycle self…

....

....

....

....

....

....

....

....

Your Cycle Wheel

Start date:

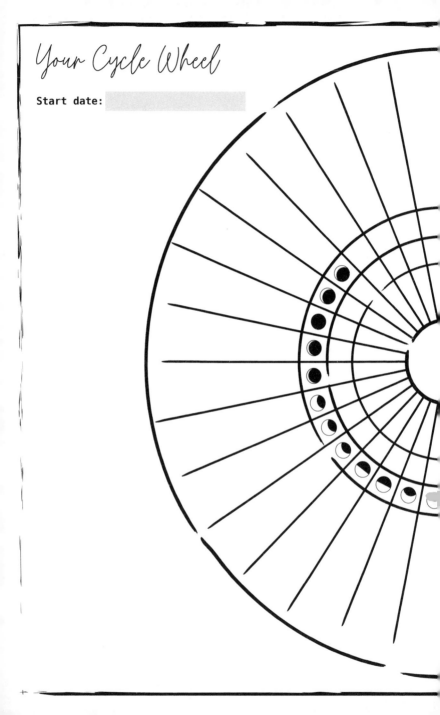

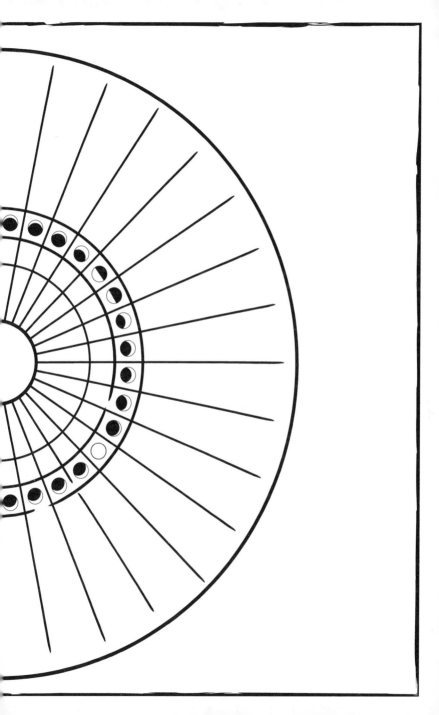

Date: Cycle day:

Cycle phase: Moon phase:

Day/planetary energy: Sun sign:

The Feels

_____

_____

_____

Self-sourcing

_____

_____

_____

Heart Riffs

_____

_____

_____

_____

Date: Cycle day:

Cycle phase: Moon phase:

Day/planetary energy: Sun sign:

The Feels

_____

_____

_____

Self-sourcing

_____

_____

_____

Heart Riffs

_____

_____

_____

_____

Date: Cycle day:
Cycle phase: Moon phase:
Day/planetary energy: Sun sign:

The Feels 🫶

_____
_____
_____

Self-sourcing 🧘

_____
_____
_____

Heart Riffs ✍

_____
_____
_____

Date: Cycle day:
Cycle phase: Moon phase:
Day/planetary energy: Sun sign:

The Feels 🫶

_____
_____
_____

Self-sourcing 🧘

_____
_____
_____

Heart Riffs ✍

_____
_____
_____

Date: Cycle day:

Cycle phase: Moon phase:

Day/planetary energy: Sun sign:

The Feels

_____

_____

_____

Self-sourcing

_____

_____

_____

Heart Riffs

_____

_____

_____

Date: Cycle day:

Cycle phase: Moon phase:

Day/planetary energy: Sun sign:

The Feels

_____

_____

_____

Self-sourcing

_____

_____

_____

Heart Riffs

_____

_____

_____

Date: Cycle day:

Cycle phase: Moon phase:

Day/planetary energy: Sun sign:

The Feels 🫶

_____

_____

_____

_____

Self-sourcing 🧘

_____

_____

_____

_____

Heart Riffs ✍️

_____

_____

_____

_____

Date: Cycle day:

Cycle phase: Moon phase:

Day/planetary energy: Sun sign:

The Feels 🫶

_____

_____

_____

_____

Self-sourcing 🧘

_____

_____

_____

_____

Heart Riffs ✍️

_____

_____

_____

_____

Date: Cycle day:

Cycle phase: Moon phase:

Day/planetary energy: Sun sign:

The Feels 🤲

_____

_____

_____

Self-sourcing 🧘

_____

_____

_____

Heart Riffs ✍️

_____

_____

_____

_____

Date: Cycle day:

Cycle phase: Moon phase:

Day/planetary energy: Sun sign:

The Feels 🤲

_____

_____

_____

Self-sourcing 🧘

_____

_____

_____

Heart Riffs ✍️

_____

_____

_____

_____

Date: _____ Cycle day: _____

Cycle phase: _____ Moon phase: _____

Day/planetary energy: _____ Sun sign: _____

The Feels

_____

_____

_____

Self-sourcing

_____

_____

_____

Heart Riffs

_____

_____

_____

_____

Date: _____ Cycle day: _____

Cycle phase: _____ Moon phase: _____

Day/planetary energy: _____ Sun sign: _____

The Feels

_____

_____

_____

Self-sourcing

_____

_____

_____

Heart Riffs

_____

_____

_____

_____

Date: _____   Cycle day: _____

Cycle phase: _____   Moon phase: _____

Day/planetary energy: _____   Sun sign: _____

The Feels 🤲

_____

_____

_____

_____

Self-sourcing 🧘

_____

_____

_____

_____

Heart Riffs ✍️

_____

_____

_____

_____

Date: _____   Cycle day: _____

Cycle phase: _____   Moon phase: _____

Day/planetary energy: _____   Sun sign: _____

The Feels 🤲

_____

_____

_____

_____

Self-sourcing 🧘

_____

_____

_____

_____

Heart Riffs ✍️

_____

_____

_____

_____

Date: _____   Cycle day: _____

Cycle phase: _____   Moon phase: _____

Day/planetary energy: _____   Sun sign: _____

The Feels 🤲

_____

_____

_____

_____

Self-sourcing 🧘

_____

_____

_____

_____

Heart Riffs ✍

_____

_____

_____

_____

Date: _____   Cycle day: _____

Cycle phase: _____   Moon phase: _____

Day/planetary energy: _____   Sun sign: _____

The Feels 🤲

_____

_____

_____

_____

Self-sourcing 🧘

_____

_____

_____

_____

Heart Riffs ✍

_____

_____

_____

_____

Date: _____   Cycle day: _____

Cycle phase: _____   Moon phase: _____

Day/planetary energy: _____   Sun sign: _____

The Feels 🤲

_____

_____

_____

_____

Self-sourcing 🧘

_____

_____

_____

_____

Heart Riffs ✍️

_____

_____

_____

_____

Date: _____   Cycle day: _____

Cycle phase: _____   Moon phase: _____

Day/planetary energy: _____   Sun sign: _____

The Feels 🤲

_____

_____

_____

_____

Self-sourcing 🧘

_____

_____

_____

_____

Heart Riffs ✍️

_____

_____

_____

_____

Date: Cycle day:

Cycle phase: Moon phase:

Day/planetary energy: Sun sign:

The Feels 🫶

_____

_____

_____

_____

Self-sourcing 🧘

_____

_____

_____

Heart Riffs ✍️

_____

_____

_____

_____

Date: Cycle day:

Cycle phase: Moon phase:

Day/planetary energy: Sun sign:

The Feels 🫶

_____

_____

_____

_____

Self-sourcing 🧘

_____

_____

_____

Heart Riffs ✍️

_____

_____

_____

_____

Date: ⬚ Cycle day: ⬚
Cycle phase: ⬚ Moon phase: ⬚
Day/planetary energy: ⬚ Sun sign: ⬚

The Feels 🤲

_____
_____
_____
_____

Self-sourcing 🧘

_____
_____
_____
_____

Heart Riffs ✍️

_____
_____
_____
_____

Date: ⬚ Cycle day: ⬚
Cycle phase: ⬚ Moon phase: ⬚
Day/planetary energy: ⬚ Sun sign: ⬚

The Feels 🤲

_____
_____
_____
_____

Self-sourcing 🧘

_____
_____
_____
_____

Heart Riffs ✍️

_____
_____
_____
_____

Date: _____ Cycle day: _____
Cycle phase: _____ Moon phase: _____
Day/planetary energy: _____ Sun sign: _____

The Feels ✍

_____
_____
_____
_____

Self-sourcing 🧘

_____
_____
_____
_____

Heart Riffs ✍

_____
_____
_____
_____

Date: _____ Cycle day: _____
Cycle phase: _____ Moon phase: _____
Day/planetary energy: _____ Sun sign: _____

The Feels ✍

_____
_____
_____
_____

Self-sourcing 🧘

_____
_____
_____
_____

Heart Riffs ✍

_____
_____
_____
_____

Date: _____ Cycle day: _____

Cycle phase: _____ Moon phase: _____

Day/planetary energy: _____ Sun sign: _____

The Feels 🫶

_____

_____

_____

_____

Self-sourcing 🧘

_____

_____

_____

_____

Heart Riffs ✍️

_____

_____

_____

_____

Date: _____ Cycle day: _____

Cycle phase: _____ Moon phase: _____

Day/planetary energy: _____ Sun sign: _____

The Feels 🫶

_____

_____

_____

_____

Self-sourcing 🧘

_____

_____

_____

_____

Heart Riffs ✍️

_____

_____

_____

_____

Date: _____ Cycle day: _____

Cycle phase: _____ Moon phase: _____

Day/planetary energy: _____ Sun sign: _____

The Feels 🫶

_____

_____

_____

_____

Self-sourcing 🧘

_____

_____

_____

_____

Heart Riffs ✍️

_____

_____

_____

_____

Date: _____ Cycle day: _____

Cycle phase: _____ Moon phase: _____

Day/planetary energy: _____ Sun sign: _____

The Feels 🫶

_____

_____

_____

_____

Self-sourcing 🧘

_____

_____

_____

_____

Heart Riffs ✍️

_____

_____

_____

_____

Date: Cycle day:

Cycle phase: Moon phase:

Day/planetary energy: Sun sign:

The Feels

_____

_____

_____

_____

Self-sourcing

_____

_____

_____

Heart Riffs

_____

_____

_____

_____

Date: Cycle day:

Cycle phase: Moon phase:

Day/planetary energy: Sun sign:

The Feels

_____

_____

_____

_____

Self-sourcing

_____

_____

_____

Heart Riffs

_____

_____

_____

_____

Date: _____ Cycle day: _____

Cycle phase: _____ Moon phase: _____

Day/planetary energy: _____ Sun sign: _____

The Feels 🫶

_____

_____

_____

_____

Self-sourcing 🧘

_____

_____

_____

_____

Heart Riffs ✍️

_____

_____

_____

_____

Date: _____ Cycle day: _____

Cycle phase: _____ Moon phase: _____

Day/planetary energy: _____ Sun sign: _____

The Feels 🫶

_____

_____

_____

_____

Self-sourcing 🧘

_____

_____

_____

_____

Heart Riffs ✍️

_____

_____

_____

_____

Reflect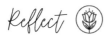

Which cycle days were most positive?

....

....

....

....

....

....

....

Which were most challenging?

....

....

....

....

....

....

....

....

What patterns are unfolding?

....

....

....

....

....

....

....

Notes for your next-cycle self…

....

....

....

....

....

....

....

....

Your Cycle Wheel

Start date:

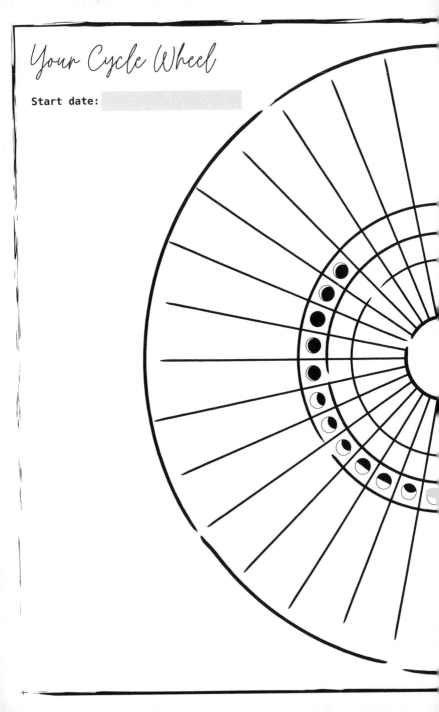

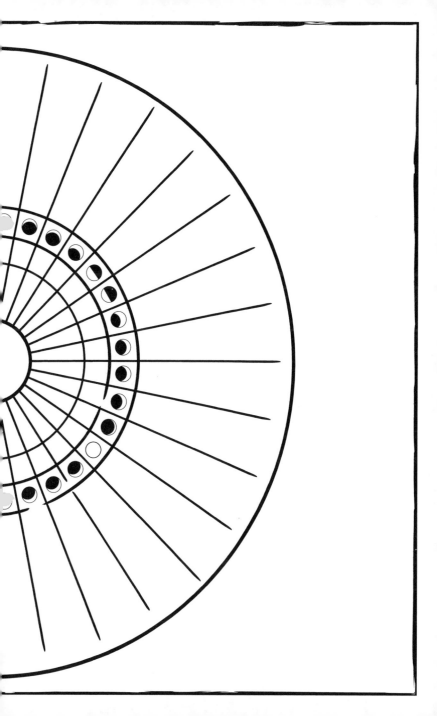

Date: _____ Cycle day: _____

Cycle phase: _____ Moon phase: _____

Day/planetary energy: _____ Sun sign: _____

The Feels 🫶

_____

_____

_____

_____

Self-sourcing 🧘

_____

_____

_____

_____

Heart Riffs ✍️

_____

_____

_____

_____

Date: _____ Cycle day: _____

Cycle phase: _____ Moon phase: _____

Day/planetary energy: _____ Sun sign: _____

The Feels 🫶

_____

_____

_____

_____

Self-sourcing 🧘

_____

_____

_____

_____

Heart Riffs ✍️

_____

_____

_____

_____

Date: _____ Cycle day: _____
Cycle phase: _____ Moon phase: _____
Day/planetary energy: _____ Sun sign: _____

The Feels ✋

_____
_____
_____
_____

Self-sourcing 🧘

_____
_____
_____

Heart Riffs ✍️

_____
_____
_____
_____

Date: _____ Cycle day: _____
Cycle phase: _____ Moon phase: _____
Day/planetary energy: _____ Sun sign: _____

The Feels ✋

_____
_____
_____
_____

Self-sourcing 🧘

_____
_____
_____

Heart Riffs ✍️

_____
_____
_____
_____

Date: _____ Cycle day: _____

Cycle phase: _____ Moon phase: _____

Day/planetary energy: _____ Sun sign: _____

The Feels 🤟

_____
_____
_____

Self-sourcing 🧘

_____
_____
_____

Heart Riffs ✍️

_____
_____
_____
_____

Date: _____ Cycle day: _____

Cycle phase: _____ Moon phase: _____

Day/planetary energy: _____ Sun sign: _____

The Feels 🤟

_____
_____
_____

Self-sourcing 🧘

_____
_____
_____

Heart Riffs ✍️

_____
_____
_____

Date: _____ Cycle day: _____

Cycle phase: _____ Moon phase: _____

Day/planetary energy: _____ Sun sign: _____

The Feels 🫶

_____

_____

_____

_____

Self-sourcing 🧘

_____

_____

_____

Heart Riffs ✍️

_____

_____

_____

_____

Date: _____ Cycle day: _____

Cycle phase: _____ Moon phase: _____

Day/planetary energy: _____ Sun sign: _____

The Feels 🫶

_____

_____

_____

_____

Self-sourcing 🧘

_____

_____

_____

Heart Riffs ✍️

_____

_____

_____

_____

Date: Cycle day:
Cycle phase: Moon phase:
Day/planetary energy: Sun sign:

The Feels 🤟

_____
_____
_____
_____

Self-sourcing 🧘

_____
_____
_____
_____

Heart Riffs ✍️

_____
_____
_____
_____

Date: Cycle day:
Cycle phase: Moon phase:
Day/planetary energy: Sun sign:

The Feels 🤟

_____
_____
_____
_____

Self-sourcing 🧘

_____
_____
_____
_____

Heart Riffs ✍️

_____
_____
_____
_____

Date: _____ Cycle day: _____

Cycle phase: _____ Moon phase: _____

Day/planetary energy: _____ Sun sign: _____

The Feels 🤲

_____

_____

_____

_____

Self-sourcing 🧘

_____

_____

_____

_____

Heart Riffs ✍️

_____

_____

_____

_____

Date: _____ Cycle day: _____

Cycle phase: _____ Moon phase: _____

Day/planetary energy: _____ Sun sign: _____

The Feels 🤲

_____

_____

_____

_____

Self-sourcing 🧘

_____

_____

_____

_____

Heart Riffs ✍️

_____

_____

_____

_____

Date: _____   Cycle day: _____

Cycle phase: _____   Moon phase: _____

Day/planetary energy: _____   Sun sign: _____

The Feels 🫶

_____

_____

_____

Self-sourcing 🧘

_____

_____

_____

Heart Riffs ✍️

_____

_____

_____

_____

Date: _____   Cycle day: _____

Cycle phase: _____   Moon phase: _____

Day/planetary energy: _____   Sun sign: _____

The Feels 🫶

_____

_____

_____

Self-sourcing 🧘

_____

_____

_____

Heart Riffs ✍️

_____

_____

_____

Date: _____ Cycle day: _____

Cycle phase: _____ Moon phase: _____

Day/planetary energy: _____ Sun sign: _____

The Feels ⊛

_____

_____

_____

Self-sourcing ⊛

_____

_____

_____

Heart Riffs ⊛

_____

_____

_____

Date: _____ Cycle day: _____

Cycle phase: _____ Moon phase: _____

Day/planetary energy: _____ Sun sign: _____

The Feels ⊛

_____

_____

_____

Self-sourcing ⊛

_____

_____

_____

Heart Riffs ⊛

_____

_____

_____

Date: Cycle day:
Cycle phase: Moon phase:
Day/planetary energy: Sun sign:

The Feels 🤟

Self-sourcing 🧘

Heart Riffs ✍

Date: Cycle day:
Cycle phase: Moon phase:
Day/planetary energy: Sun sign:

The Feels 🤟

Self-sourcing 🧘

Heart Riffs ✍

Date: _____ Cycle day: _____
Cycle phase: _____ Moon phase: _____
Day/planetary energy: _____ Sun sign: _____

The Feels

_____
_____
_____
_____

Self-sourcing

_____
_____
_____
_____

Heart Riffs

_____
_____
_____
_____

Date: _____ Cycle day: _____
Cycle phase: _____ Moon phase: _____
Day/planetary energy: _____ Sun sign: _____

The Feels

_____
_____
_____
_____

Self-sourcing

_____
_____
_____
_____

Heart Riffs

_____
_____
_____
_____

Date: Cycle day:

Cycle phase: Moon phase:

Day/planetary energy: Sun sign:

The Feels

_____

_____

_____

Self-sourcing

_____

_____

_____

Heart Riffs

_____

_____

_____

_____

Date: Cycle day:

Cycle phase: Moon phase:

Day/planetary energy: Sun sign:

The Feels

_____

_____

_____

Self-sourcing

_____

_____

_____

Heart Riffs

_____

_____

_____

Date: Cycle day:

Cycle phase: Moon phase:

Day/planetary energy: Sun sign:

The Feels

_____
_____
_____
_____

Self-sourcing

_____
_____
_____
_____

Heart Riffs

_____
_____
_____
_____

Date: Cycle day:

Cycle phase: Moon phase:

Day/planetary energy: Sun sign:

The Feels

_____
_____
_____
_____

Self-sourcing

_____
_____
_____
_____

Heart Riffs

_____
_____
_____
_____

Date: Cycle day:
Cycle phase: Moon phase:
Day/planetary energy: Sun sign:

The Feels 🫶

_____
_____
_____
_____

Self-sourcing 🧘

_____
_____
_____
_____

Heart Riffs ✍️

_____
_____
_____
_____

Date: Cycle day:
Cycle phase: Moon phase:
Day/planetary energy: Sun sign:

The Feels 🫶

_____
_____
_____
_____

Self-sourcing 🧘

_____
_____
_____
_____

Heart Riffs ✍️

_____
_____
_____
_____

Date: Cycle day:

Cycle phase: Moon phase:

Day/planetary energy: Sun sign:

The Feels

Self-sourcing

Heart Riffs

Date: Cycle day:

Cycle phase: Moon phase:

Day/planetary energy: Sun sign:

The Feels

Self-sourcing

Heart Riffs

Date: _____ Cycle day: _____
Cycle phase: _____ Moon phase: _____
Day/planetary energy: _____ Sun sign: _____

The Feels 🫶

_____
_____
_____
_____

Self-sourcing 🧘

_____
_____
_____
_____

Heart Riffs ✍️

_____
_____
_____
_____

Date: _____ Cycle day: _____
Cycle phase: _____ Moon phase: _____
Day/planetary energy: _____ Sun sign: _____

The Feels 🫶

_____
_____
_____
_____

Self-sourcing 🧘

_____
_____
_____
_____

Heart Riffs ✍️

_____
_____
_____
_____

Date: _____ Cycle day: _____
Cycle phase: _____ Moon phase: _____
Day/planetary energy: _____ Sun sign: _____

The Feels 🫶

_____
_____
_____
_____

Self-sourcing 🧘

_____
_____
_____

Heart Riffs ✍️

_____
_____
_____
_____

Date: _____ Cycle day: _____
Cycle phase: _____ Moon phase: _____
Day/planetary energy: _____ Sun sign: _____

The Feels 🫶

_____
_____
_____
_____

Self-sourcing 🧘

_____
_____
_____

Heart Riffs ✍️

_____
_____
_____
_____

Reflect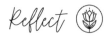

Which cycle days were most positive?

_____

_____

_____

_____

_____

_____

_____

Which were most challenging?

_____

_____

_____

_____

_____

_____

_____

_____

What patterns are unfolding?

Notes for your next-cycle self…

Your Cycle Wheel

Start date:

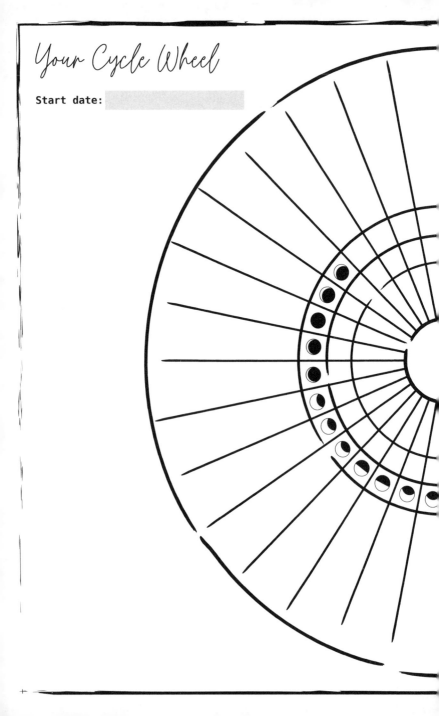

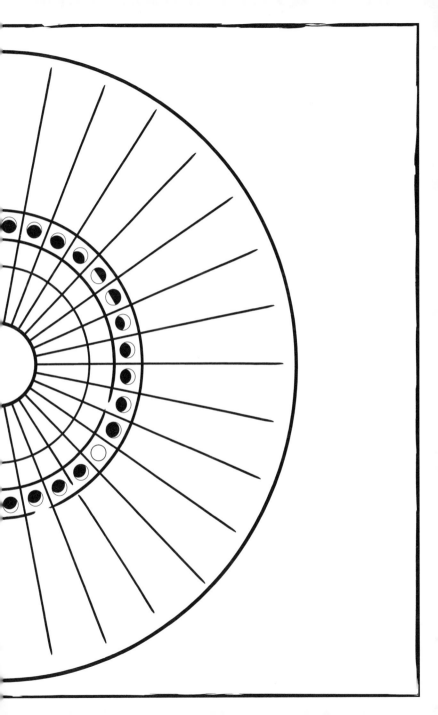

Date: Cycle day:

Cycle phase: Moon phase:

Day/planetary energy: Sun sign:

The Feels

Self-sourcing

Heart Riffs

Date: Cycle day:

Cycle phase: Moon phase:

Day/planetary energy: Sun sign:

The Feels

Self-sourcing

Heart Riffs

Date: Cycle day:

Cycle phase: Moon phase:

Day/planetary energy: Sun sign:

The Feels

Self-sourcing

Heart Riffs

Date: Cycle day:

Cycle phase: Moon phase:

Day/planetary energy: Sun sign:

The Feels

Self-sourcing

Heart Riffs

Date: _____ Cycle day: _____

Cycle phase: _____ Moon phase: _____

Day/planetary energy: _____ Sun sign: _____

The Feels 🫶

_____
_____
_____
_____

Self-sourcing 🧘

_____
_____
_____
_____

Heart Riffs ✍️

_____
_____
_____
_____

Date: _____ Cycle day: _____

Cycle phase: _____ Moon phase: _____

Day/planetary energy: _____ Sun sign: _____

The Feels 🫶

_____
_____
_____
_____

Self-sourcing 🧘

_____
_____
_____
_____

Heart Riffs ✍️

_____
_____
_____
_____

Date: _____   Cycle day: _____

Cycle phase: _____   Moon phase: _____

Day/planetary energy: _____   Sun sign: _____

The Feels 🤲

_____

_____

_____

_____

Self-sourcing 🧘

_____

_____

_____

_____

Heart Riffs ✍️

_____

_____

_____

_____

Date: _____   Cycle day: _____

Cycle phase: _____   Moon phase: _____

Day/planetary energy: _____   Sun sign: _____

The Feels 🤲

_____

_____

_____

_____

Self-sourcing 🧘

_____

_____

_____

_____

Heart Riffs ✍️

_____

_____

_____

_____

Date: _____ Cycle day: _____

Cycle phase: _____ Moon phase: _____

Day/planetary energy: _____ Sun sign: _____

The Feels ✋

_____

_____

_____

Self-sourcing 🧘

_____

_____

_____

Heart Riffs ✍

_____

_____

_____

_____

Date: _____ Cycle day: _____

Cycle phase: _____ Moon phase: _____

Day/planetary energy: _____ Sun sign: _____

The Feels ✋

_____

_____

_____

Self-sourcing 🧘

_____

_____

_____

Heart Riffs ✍

_____

_____

_____

_____

Date: Cycle day:

Cycle phase: Moon phase:

Day/planetary energy: Sun sign:

The Feels

_____

_____

_____

_____

Self-sourcing

_____

_____

_____

_____

Heart Riffs

_____

_____

_____

_____

Date: Cycle day:

Cycle phase: Moon phase:

Day/planetary energy: Sun sign:

The Feels

_____

_____

_____

_____

Self-sourcing

_____

_____

_____

_____

Heart Riffs

_____

_____

_____

_____

Date: Cycle day:

Cycle phase: Moon phase:

Day/planetary energy: Sun sign:

The Feels

Self-sourcing

Heart Riffs

Date: Cycle day:

Cycle phase: Moon phase:

Day/planetary energy: Sun sign:

The Feels

Self-sourcing

Heart Riffs

Date: _____ Cycle day: _____

Cycle phase: _____ Moon phase: _____

Day/planetary energy: _____ Sun sign: _____

The Feels 🫶

_____

_____

_____

_____

Self-sourcing 🧘

_____

_____

_____

Heart Riffs ✍️

_____

_____

_____

_____

Date: _____ Cycle day: _____

Cycle phase: _____ Moon phase: _____

Day/planetary energy: _____ Sun sign: _____

The Feels 🫶

_____

_____

_____

_____

Self-sourcing 🧘

_____

_____

_____

Heart Riffs ✍️

_____

_____

_____

Date: ＿＿＿＿＿＿＿＿＿＿＿＿＿ Cycle day: ＿＿＿＿＿＿＿＿

Cycle phase: ＿＿＿＿＿＿＿＿ Moon phase: ＿＿＿＿＿＿＿

Day/planetary energy: ＿＿＿＿＿＿＿ Sun sign: ＿＿＿＿＿＿

The Feels

＿＿＿＿＿＿＿＿＿＿＿＿＿＿＿＿＿＿＿＿＿＿＿＿＿＿＿＿＿＿＿＿

＿＿＿＿＿＿＿＿＿＿＿＿＿＿＿＿＿＿＿＿＿＿＿＿＿＿＿＿＿＿＿＿

＿＿＿＿＿＿＿＿＿＿＿＿＿＿＿＿＿＿＿＿＿＿＿＿＿＿＿＿＿＿＿＿

Self-sourcing

＿＿＿＿＿＿＿＿＿＿＿＿＿＿＿＿＿＿＿＿＿＿＿＿＿＿＿＿＿＿＿＿

＿＿＿＿＿＿＿＿＿＿＿＿＿＿＿＿＿＿＿＿＿＿＿＿＿＿＿＿＿＿＿＿

＿＿＿＿＿＿＿＿＿＿＿＿＿＿＿＿＿＿＿＿＿＿＿＿＿＿＿＿＿＿＿＿

Heart Riffs

＿＿＿＿＿＿＿＿＿＿＿＿＿＿＿＿＿＿＿＿＿＿＿＿＿＿＿＿＿＿＿＿

＿＿＿＿＿＿＿＿＿＿＿＿＿＿＿＿＿＿＿＿＿＿＿＿＿＿＿＿＿＿＿＿

＿＿＿＿＿＿＿＿＿＿＿＿＿＿＿＿＿＿＿＿＿＿＿＿＿＿＿＿＿＿＿＿

＿＿＿＿＿＿＿＿＿＿＿＿＿＿＿＿＿＿＿＿＿＿＿＿＿＿＿＿＿＿＿＿

Date: ＿＿＿＿＿＿＿＿＿＿＿＿＿ Cycle day: ＿＿＿＿＿＿＿＿

Cycle phase: ＿＿＿＿＿＿＿＿ Moon phase: ＿＿＿＿＿＿＿

Day/planetary energy: ＿＿＿＿＿＿＿ Sun sign: ＿＿＿＿＿＿

The Feels

＿＿＿＿＿＿＿＿＿＿＿＿＿＿＿＿＿＿＿＿＿＿＿＿＿＿＿＿＿＿＿＿

＿＿＿＿＿＿＿＿＿＿＿＿＿＿＿＿＿＿＿＿＿＿＿＿＿＿＿＿＿＿＿＿

＿＿＿＿＿＿＿＿＿＿＿＿＿＿＿＿＿＿＿＿＿＿＿＿＿＿＿＿＿＿＿＿

Self-sourcing

＿＿＿＿＿＿＿＿＿＿＿＿＿＿＿＿＿＿＿＿＿＿＿＿＿＿＿＿＿＿＿＿

＿＿＿＿＿＿＿＿＿＿＿＿＿＿＿＿＿＿＿＿＿＿＿＿＿＿＿＿＿＿＿＿

＿＿＿＿＿＿＿＿＿＿＿＿＿＿＿＿＿＿＿＿＿＿＿＿＿＿＿＿＿＿＿＿

Heart Riffs

＿＿＿＿＿＿＿＿＿＿＿＿＿＿＿＿＿＿＿＿＿＿＿＿＿＿＿＿＿＿＿＿

＿＿＿＿＿＿＿＿＿＿＿＿＿＿＿＿＿＿＿＿＿＿＿＿＿＿＿＿＿＿＿＿

＿＿＿＿＿＿＿＿＿＿＿＿＿＿＿＿＿＿＿＿＿＿＿＿＿＿＿＿＿＿＿＿

＿＿＿＿＿＿＿＿＿＿＿＿＿＿＿＿＿＿＿＿＿＿＿＿＿＿＿＿＿＿＿＿

Date: _____ Cycle day: _____

Cycle phase: _____ Moon phase: _____

Day/planetary energy: _____ Sun sign: _____

The Feels ✋

_____

_____

_____

_____

Self-sourcing 🧘

_____

_____

_____

_____

Heart Riffs ✍

_____

_____

_____

_____

Date: _____ Cycle day: _____

Cycle phase: _____ Moon phase: _____

Day/planetary energy: _____ Sun sign: _____

The Feels ✋

_____

_____

_____

_____

Self-sourcing 🧘

_____

_____

_____

_____

Heart Riffs ✍

_____

_____

_____

_____

Date: _____ Cycle day: _____

Cycle phase: _____ Moon phase: _____

Day/planetary energy: _____ Sun sign: _____

The Feels 🫶

_____

_____

_____

_____

Self-sourcing 🧘

_____

_____

_____

Heart Riffs ✍️

_____

_____

_____

_____

Date: _____ Cycle day: _____

Cycle phase: _____ Moon phase: _____

Day/planetary energy: _____ Sun sign: _____

The Feels 🫶

_____

_____

_____

_____

Self-sourcing 🧘

_____

_____

_____

Heart Riffs ✍️

_____

_____

_____

_____

Date: _____ Cycle day: _____

Cycle phase: _____ Moon phase: _____

Day/planetary energy: _____ Sun sign: _____

The Feels 🫶

_____

_____

_____

Self-sourcing 🧘

_____

_____

_____

Heart Riffs ✍️

_____

_____

_____

Date: _____ Cycle day: _____

Cycle phase: _____ Moon phase: _____

Day/planetary energy: _____ Sun sign: _____

The Feels 🫶

_____

_____

_____

Self-sourcing 🧘

_____

_____

_____

Heart Riffs ✍️

_____

_____

_____

Date: _____ Cycle day: _____
Cycle phase: _____ Moon phase: _____
Day/planetary energy: _____ Sun sign: _____

The Feels 🤟

_____
_____
_____

Self-sourcing 🧘

_____
_____
_____

Heart Riffs ✍

_____
_____
_____

Date: _____ Cycle day: _____
Cycle phase: _____ Moon phase: _____
Day/planetary energy: _____ Sun sign: _____

The Feels 🤟

_____
_____
_____

Self-sourcing 🧘

_____
_____
_____

Heart Riffs ✍

_____
_____
_____

Date: _____ Cycle day: _____

Cycle phase: _____ Moon phase: _____

Day/planetary energy: _____ Sun sign: _____

The Feels 🫶

_____
_____
_____
_____

Self-sourcing 🧘

_____
_____
_____
_____

Heart Riffs ✍️

_____
_____
_____
_____

Date: _____ Cycle day: _____

Cycle phase: _____ Moon phase: _____

Day/planetary energy: _____ Sun sign: _____

The Feels 🫶

_____
_____
_____
_____

Self-sourcing 🧘

_____
_____
_____
_____

Heart Riffs ✍️

_____
_____
_____
_____

Date: _____ Cycle day: _____
Cycle phase: _____ Moon phase: _____
Day/planetary energy: _____ Sun sign: _____

The Feels ✋

_____
_____
_____
_____

Self-sourcing 🧘

_____
_____
_____
_____

Heart Riffs ✍

_____
_____
_____
_____

Date: _____ Cycle day: _____
Cycle phase: _____ Moon phase: _____
Day/planetary energy: _____ Sun sign: _____

The Feels ✋

_____
_____
_____
_____

Self-sourcing 🧘

_____
_____
_____
_____

Heart Riffs ✍

_____
_____
_____
_____

Date: Cycle day:

Cycle phase: Moon phase:

Day/planetary energy: Sun sign:

The Feels 🫶

Self-sourcing 🧘

Heart Riffs ✍️

Date: Cycle day:

Cycle phase: Moon phase:

Day/planetary energy: Sun sign:

The Feels 🫶

Self-sourcing 🧘

Heart Riffs ✍️

Reflect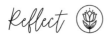

Which cycle days were most positive?

_____

_____

_____

_____

_____

_____

_____

Which were most challenging?

_____

_____

_____

_____

_____

_____

_____

_____

_____

What patterns are unfolding?

Notes for your next-cycle self…

Your Cycle Wheel

Start date:

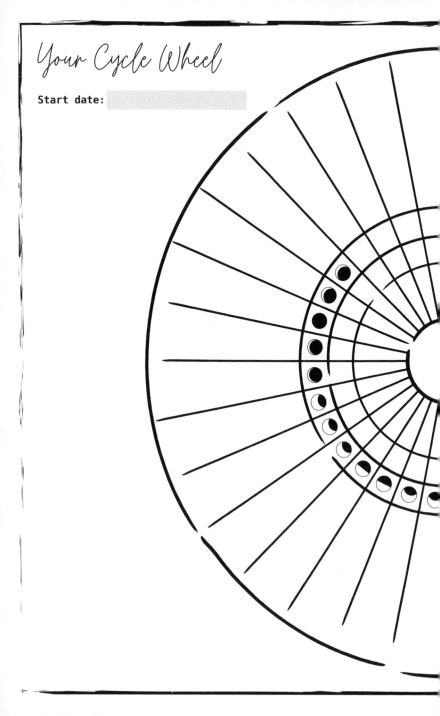

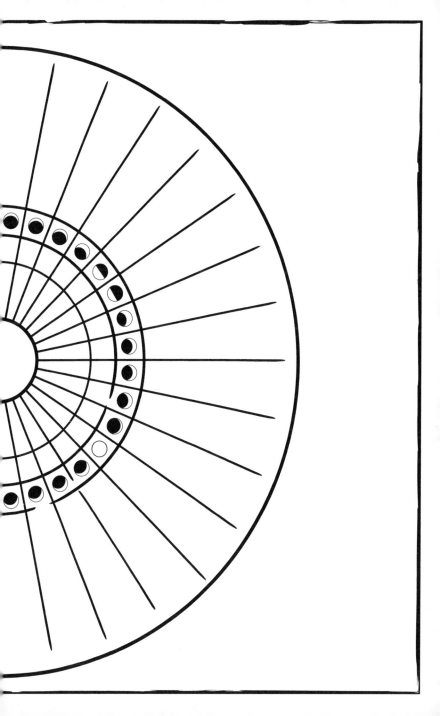

Date: _____ Cycle day: _____

Cycle phase: _____ Moon phase: _____

Day/planetary energy: _____ Sun sign: _____

The Feels 🫶

_____

_____

_____

_____

Self-sourcing 🧘

_____

_____

_____

_____

Heart Riffs ✍️

_____

_____

_____

_____

Date: _____ Cycle day: _____

Cycle phase: _____ Moon phase: _____

Day/planetary energy: _____ Sun sign: _____

The Feels 🫶

_____

_____

_____

_____

Self-sourcing 🧘

_____

_____

_____

_____

Heart Riffs ✍️

_____

_____

_____

_____

Date: _____ Cycle day: _____

Cycle phase: _____ Moon phase: _____

Day/planetary energy: _____ Sun sign: _____

The Feels 🤲

_____

_____

_____

_____

Self-sourcing 🧘

_____

_____

_____

_____

Heart Riffs ✍️

_____

_____

_____

_____

Date: _____ Cycle day: _____

Cycle phase: _____ Moon phase: _____

Day/planetary energy: _____ Sun sign: _____

The Feels 🤲

_____

_____

_____

_____

Self-sourcing 🧘

_____

_____

_____

_____

Heart Riffs ✍️

_____

_____

_____

_____

Date: _____   Cycle day: _____
Cycle phase: _____   Moon phase: _____
Day/planetary energy: _____   Sun sign: _____

The Feels ✋

_____
_____
_____
_____

Self-sourcing 🧘

_____
_____
_____
_____

Heart Riffs ✍

_____
_____
_____
_____

Date: _____   Cycle day: _____
Cycle phase: _____   Moon phase: _____
Day/planetary energy: _____   Sun sign: _____

The Feels ✋

_____
_____
_____
_____

Self-sourcing 🧘

_____
_____
_____
_____

Heart Riffs ✍

_____
_____
_____
_____

Date: _____ Cycle day: _____

Cycle phase: _____ Moon phase: _____

Day/planetary energy: _____ Sun sign: _____

The Feels 🫶

_____

_____

_____

_____

Self-sourcing 🧘

_____

_____

_____

Heart Riffs ✍️

_____

_____

_____

_____

Date: _____ Cycle day: _____

Cycle phase: _____ Moon phase: _____

Day/planetary energy: _____ Sun sign: _____

The Feels 🫶

_____

_____

_____

_____

Self-sourcing 🧘

_____

_____

_____

Heart Riffs ✍️

_____

_____

_____

_____

Date: _____ Cycle day: _____

Cycle phase: _____ Moon phase: _____

Day/planetary energy: _____ Sun sign: _____

The Feels ✋

_____

_____

_____

Self-sourcing 🧘

_____

_____

_____

Heart Riffs ✍

_____

_____

_____

_____

Date: _____ Cycle day: _____

Cycle phase: _____ Moon phase: _____

Day/planetary energy: _____ Sun sign: _____

The Feels ✋

_____

_____

_____

Self-sourcing 🧘

_____

_____

_____

Heart Riffs ✍

_____

_____

_____

_____

Date: _____ Cycle day: _____

Cycle phase: _____ Moon phase: _____

Day/planetary energy: _____ Sun sign: _____

The Feels ✋

_____

_____

_____

Self-sourcing 🧘

_____

_____

_____

Heart Riffs ✍

_____

_____

_____

Date: _____ Cycle day: _____

Cycle phase: _____ Moon phase: _____

Day/planetary energy: _____ Sun sign: _____

The Feels ✋

_____

_____

_____

Self-sourcing 🧘

_____

_____

_____

Heart Riffs ✍

_____

_____

_____

Date: Cycle day:

Cycle phase: Moon phase:

Day/planetary energy: Sun sign:

The Feels

_____
_____
_____
_____

Self-sourcing

_____
_____
_____
_____

Heart Riffs

_____
_____
_____
_____

Date: Cycle day:

Cycle phase: Moon phase:

Day/planetary energy: Sun sign:

The Feels

_____
_____
_____
_____

Self-sourcing

_____
_____
_____
_____

Heart Riffs

_____
_____
_____
_____

Date: _____ Cycle day: _____
Cycle phase: _____ Moon phase: _____
Day/planetary energy: _____ Sun sign: _____

The Feels 🫶

_____
_____
_____

Self-sourcing 🧘

_____
_____
_____

Heart Riffs ✍️

_____
_____
_____
_____

Date: _____ Cycle day: _____
Cycle phase: _____ Moon phase: _____
Day/planetary energy: _____ Sun sign: _____

The Feels 🫶

_____
_____
_____

Self-sourcing 🧘

_____
_____
_____

Heart Riffs ✍️

_____
_____
_____

Date: Cycle day:

Cycle phase: Moon phase:

Day/planetary energy: Sun sign:

The Feels 🫶

Self-sourcing 🧘

Heart Riffs ✍️

Date: Cycle day:

Cycle phase: Moon phase:

Day/planetary energy: Sun sign:

The Feels 🫶

Self-sourcing 🧘

Heart Riffs ✍️

Date: Cycle day:

Cycle phase: Moon phase:

Day/planetary energy: Sun sign:

The Feels

Self-sourcing

Heart Riffs

Date: Cycle day:

Cycle phase: Moon phase:

Day/planetary energy: Sun sign:

The Feels

Self-sourcing

Heart Riffs

Date: _____ Cycle day: _____
Cycle phase: _____ Moon phase: _____
Day/planetary energy: _____ Sun sign: _____

The Feels 🤲

_____
_____
_____
_____

Self-sourcing 🧘

_____
_____
_____
_____

Heart Riffs ✍️

_____
_____
_____
_____

Date: _____ Cycle day: _____
Cycle phase: _____ Moon phase: _____
Day/planetary energy: _____ Sun sign: _____

The Feels 🤲

_____
_____
_____
_____

Self-sourcing 🧘

_____
_____
_____
_____

Heart Riffs ✍️

_____
_____
_____
_____

Date: ⬚⬚⬚⬚⬚⬚⬚⬚⬚⬚⬚⬚ Cycle day: ⬚⬚⬚⬚⬚⬚⬚⬚⬚

Cycle phase: ⬚⬚⬚⬚⬚⬚⬚⬚ Moon phase: ⬚⬚⬚⬚⬚⬚⬚⬚⬚⬚

Day/planetary energy: ⬚⬚⬚⬚⬚⬚⬚⬚⬚⬚⬚⬚ Sun sign: ⬚⬚⬚⬚⬚⬚⬚

The Feels 🤲

_____

_____

_____

Self-sourcing 🧘

_____

_____

_____

Heart Riffs ✍️

_____

_____

_____

Date: ⬚⬚⬚⬚⬚⬚⬚⬚⬚⬚⬚⬚ Cycle day: ⬚⬚⬚⬚⬚⬚⬚⬚⬚

Cycle phase: ⬚⬚⬚⬚⬚⬚⬚⬚ Moon phase: ⬚⬚⬚⬚⬚⬚⬚⬚⬚⬚

Day/planetary energy: ⬚⬚⬚⬚⬚⬚⬚⬚⬚⬚⬚⬚ Sun sign: ⬚⬚⬚⬚⬚⬚⬚

The Feels 🤲

_____

_____

_____

Self-sourcing 🧘

_____

_____

_____

Heart Riffs ✍️

_____

_____

_____

Date: _____ Cycle day: _____

Cycle phase: _____ Moon phase: _____

Day/planetary energy: _____ Sun sign: _____

The Feels 🤲

_____

_____

_____

Self-sourcing 🧘

_____

_____

_____

Heart Riffs ✍️

_____

_____

_____

_____

Date: _____ Cycle day: _____

Cycle phase: _____ Moon phase: _____

Day/planetary energy: _____ Sun sign: _____

The Feels 🤲

_____

_____

_____

Self-sourcing 🧘

_____

_____

_____

Heart Riffs ✍️

_____

_____

_____

_____

Date: Cycle day:

Cycle phase: Moon phase:

Day/planetary energy: Sun sign:

The Feels

Self-sourcing

Heart Riffs

Date: Cycle day:

Cycle phase: Moon phase:

Day/planetary energy: Sun sign:

The Feels

Self-sourcing

Heart Riffs

Date: Cycle day:

Cycle phase: Moon phase:

Day/planetary energy: Sun sign:

The Feels 🫶

_____

_____

_____

Self-sourcing 🧘

_____

_____

_____

Heart Riffs ✍️

_____

_____

_____

_____

Date: Cycle day:

Cycle phase: Moon phase:

Day/planetary energy: Sun sign:

The Feels 🫶

_____

_____

_____

Self-sourcing 🧘

_____

_____

_____

Heart Riffs ✍️

_____

_____

_____

_____

Date: _____ Cycle day: _____

Cycle phase: _____ Moon phase: _____

Day/planetary energy: _____ Sun sign: _____

The Feels 🤲

_____

_____

_____

_____

Self-sourcing 🧘

_____

_____

_____

_____

Heart Riffs ✍️

_____

_____

_____

_____

Date: _____ Cycle day: _____

Cycle phase: _____ Moon phase: _____

Day/planetary energy: _____ Sun sign: _____

The Feels 🤲

_____

_____

_____

_____

Self-sourcing 🧘

_____

_____

_____

_____

Heart Riffs ✍️

_____

_____

_____

_____

Reflect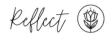

Which cycle days were most positive?

_____

_____

_____

_____

_____

_____

_____

Which were most challenging?

_____

_____

_____

_____

_____

_____

_____

_____

What patterns are unfolding?

Notes for your next-cycle self...

Okay, So What Do I Do Now?

N ow is where the work can really begin.

You've collated your cyclic intel, and potentially now have 13 cycles of personal wisdom held within these pages.

Firstly, you're bloody brilliant.

Secondly, isn't filling in your own *Red Journal* way more pleasurable than simply storing data on a phone app?!

Now, the invitation is to mine for the gold.

Your gold.

Insight and intel to the experience of being you.

If I'd been taught about this cyclic wisdom—the phases of my cycle and how to chart them—from menarche, my first bleed, I would now have a full-to-the-brim, go-to guidebook to my moods, feelings, and emotions.

I would know myself.

I would have had fewer arguments with my parents, a better understanding of my friendship dynamics with other women, and, quite frankly, I'd definitely have had a much better sex life in my twenties.

So, don't waste a single minute, get to know your flow and let the unlocking of your superpowers and your cyclic wisdom begin.

What affects your feelings and emotions, and, most importantly, when are they triggered? What cycle phase are you in when they're triggered? Where's the moon at?

Look to see if day 21, for example, evokes the same thoughts and feelings for you each month, and if so, what can you do to ease it, or make it better?

I have a gorgeous friend who highlights her bleed days in her diary and puts an "out of office" on her email saying, "Please do not disturb, I'm bleeding." And literally takes four days off. Each month.

Now, I know that's not possible for many of us—our cycle may not be so predictable, we may have work and family commitments—but imagine a day like that, or even an hour.

Day 25 is an absolute non-negotiable day off in my world. It's not a bleed day, but it's a day, as I mentioned previously, that I've identified, through charting my cycle, as a day I need to not be around people. I won't coach clients, I won't do interviews, meet with friends, go out, go online, or even answer the door, because I know that I have a tendency to kick off, get mad, scream and shout a lot. Instead of trying to push it down and repress it, I allow my Wise, Wild Woman within a day to express herself.

I have cave time: I lay out my sheepskin rug; light candles; take my journal, a good book, a flask of tea (and if the Viking is home, he'll leave me food outside the door); and I allow myself to be fully in it. Sometimes it comes and I have to hit a pillow, but more often than not, because I've created a retreat space, because I've slowed down and dropped all my responsibilities, the anger doesn't arise. Instead, I just appreciate a day to read and chill out solo.

I know this is a privilege; it's also a necessity. Taking a day during my premenstrual phase when everything is so heightened within me has saved my life. Also, just so you know, the world doesn't end if you take a day out of your schedule. I've actually found that by taking day 25 off, issues and potential dramas that would have previously unfolded because of my actions are now virtually non-existent.

Carving time out for ourselves on the days that we need it the most is the most incredible act of self-care. And self-care is NOT a luxury; it's a necessity. Make THAT your mantra as you explore your cycle.

If your cycle is more or less regular, check to see if there's a particular time in the month where you felt powerful. These are good days to know, because if they show up in the same place each month, you can start putting them to good use. Get the idea?

I want *The Red Journal* and the act of charting your cycle to help you recognize that when track your period, sync with your cycle, and unlock your monthly superpowers, you can begin to trust yourself.

You trust your body, your connection to nature and the cosmos, your cyclic nature.

You make informed decisions from a place of power.

Self-power.

Let the Red-volution commence.

Sending BIG love + appreciation to the SHE Power Collective for their support in creating *The Red Journal*, especially those who shared their big hearts, time + charting experiences with me—Nicole Carmen-Davis, Melissa Corley-Carter, Hannah Hammond, Grace Kirkby, Rebecca Lee, Sarah Steinback—I BLOODY LOVE YOU!

Want to Go Deeper?

If you want to dive deeper and explore the inner revealment and power of your menstrual cycle, you can read *Code Red: Know Your Flow, Unlock Your Monthly Superpowers, and Create a Bloody Amazing Life. Period.* (Hay House).

If you want to explore your cyclic nature and its relationship to the power that lies between your thighs, you can read *Love Your Lady Landscape: Trust Your Gut, Care For Down There and Reclaim Your Fierce and Feminine SHE Power* (Hay House).

For practical guidance, ritual and ceremony, and more insight regarding your cycle and how to work with it as monthly medicine, you can take the *Know Your Flow* online immersion that you can find at: www.thesassyshe.com/immersions

Finally, if you'd like 1-to-1 support to unlock your superpowers, understand your cyclic findings, create ritual and ceremony, or move through stuck emotions—physically and emotionally—regarding your cycle (more often than not, pain that we experience in relation to our reproductive health and menstrual cycle is a messenger for something deeper that may have been suppressed or ignored), I'm a well-woman therapist, menstrual maven and coach who offers practical, psychological, spiritual, and somatic support to women who are exploring, navigating, and healing their relationship with both their body and their cyclic nature.

Go to: www.thesassyshe.com/shesessions

ABOUT THE AUTHOR

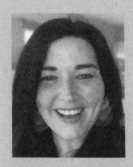

Lisa Lister, author of *Code Red, Love Your Lady Landscape* and *Witch*, is a well-woman therapist, yoga and somatic movement teacher, and menstrual maven.

Lisa offers practical, psychological, and spiritual tools, guidance, and support to women who are exploring, navigating, and healing their relationship with their body and their cyclic nature, and asking the question: what does it mean to be a woman in these "interesting" times?

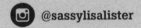 **@sassylisalister**

www.thesassyshe.com